EMERGENCIES IN OTOLARYNGOLOGY

EMERGENCIES IN OTOLARYNGOLOGY

Edited by

James Y. Suen, M.D.
Professor and Chairman
Department of Otolaryngology
 and Maxillofacial Surgery
University of Arkansas College of Medicine
Little Rock, Arkansas

Stephen J. Wetmore, M.D.
Associate Professor and Vice Chairman
Department of Otolaryngology
 and Maxillofacial Surgery
University of Arkansas College of Medicine
Chief of Otolaryngology
John L. McClellan Memorial Veterans
 Administration Medical Center
Little Rock, Arkansas

CHURCHILL LIVINGSTONE
New York, Edinburgh, London, Melbourne   1986

Library of Congress Cataloging-in-Publication Data

Emergencies in otolaryngology.
  Includes bibliographies and index.
  1. Otolaryngologic emergencies—Handbooks, manuals,
etc. I. Suen, James Y., date. II. Wetmore,
Stephen J. [DNLM: 1. Emergencies. 2. Otorhino-
laryngologic Diseases. WV 100 E53]
RF90.E44 1986   617'.51026   86-13652
ISBN 0-443-08355-X

Distributed in the United Kingdom by Churchill Livingstone,
Robert Stevenson House, 1-3 Baxter's Place, Leith Walk,
Edinburgh EH1 3AF, and by associated companies, branches,
and representatives throughout the world.

Accurate indications, adverse reactions, and dosage schedules
for drugs are provided in this book, but it is possible that they
may change. The reader is urged to review the package
information data of the manufacturers of the medications
mentioned.

Copy Editor: *Nancy Terry*
Production Designer: *Rosalie Marcus*
Production Supervisor: *Sharon Tuder*

Printed in the United States of America

First published in 1986

CONTRIBUTORS

Hassan Bashiri, D.M.D., M.S.
Assistant Professor, Department of Otolaryngology and Maxillofacial Surgery, University of Arkansas College of Medicine, Little Rock, Arkansas

Bruce Leipzig, M.D.
Private Practice in Otolaryngology, North Little Rock, Arkansas

Robert W. Seibert, M.D.
Associate Professor, Department of Otolaryngology and Maxillofacial Surgery, University of Arkansas College of Medicine; Chief of Otolaryngology, Arkansas Children's Hospital, Little Rock, Arkansas

Nancy L. Snyderman, M.D.
Assistant Professor, Department of Otolaryngology and Maxillofacial Surgery, University of Arkansas College of Medicine, Little Rock, Arkansas

James Y. Suen, M.D.
Professor and Chairman, Department of Otolaryngology and Maxillofacial Surgery, University of Arkansas College of Medicine, Little Rock, Arkansas

Stephen J. Wetmore, M.D.
Associate Professor and Vice Chairman, Department of Otolaryngology and Maxillofacial Surgery, University of Arkansas College of Medicine; Chief of Otolaryngology, John L. McClellan Memorial Veterans Administration Medical Center, Little Rock, Arkansas

PREFACE

The purpose of this book is to serve as a quick and concise guide for the many types of physicians who may initially see and treat emergency problems in the field of otolaryngology–head and neck surgery. Although the emphasis is on the diagnosis and management of common problems, a list of differential diagnoses is presented in each section so that unusual problems will not be overlooked. The primary care physician will be able to diagnose and manage most of the emergencies discussed in this book; a few of the emergencies will require referral to a physician trained in otolaryngology–head and neck surgery.

The treatment of some conditions such as facial nerve paralysis and sudden sensorineural hearing loss may not seem like emergencies to most physicians, but they are urgent problems since early treatment may reverse the disorder in some cases.

We have tried to present the most up-to-date scientific data in a thorough, yet concise, easy-to-read format, so that the reader can make an intelligent choice of therapy.

James Y. Suen, M.D.
Stephen J. Wetmore, M.D.

CONTENTS

1

Trauma to the Ear

Nancy L. Snyderman ⎯⎯⎯⎯⎯⎯⎯⎯⎯⎯⎯⎯⎯⎯⎯⎯⎯

The ear presents one of the most difficult areas for the emergency room physician to diagnose and treat. It appears inaccessible and complicated, and consequently is often overlooked during a routine examination. The morbidity from missing, misdiagnosing, or mistreating a disorder of the ear can turn a simple problem into a very complicated malady.

AURICLE

Laceration

Lacerations to the auricle are usually linear, although they may be stellate and may be complicated by a significant crush injury.

I. Evaluation
   A. Anesthetize the ear with 1% lidocaine with 1:100,000 epinephrine.
   B. Thoroughly cleanse the ear with an antibacterial solution. Ether is used if grease has contaminated an injury.
   C. Foreign body debris is removed.
   D. All nonviable skin is neatly excised with great care to save as much viable tissue as possible.

II. Skin repair
   After adequate cleansing and evaluation of the wound, the tissues and skin edges are approximated.
   A. The subcutaneous tissues are sutured with 4-0 chromic suture with buried knots.
   B. The skin edges are then lightly approximated with 5-0 or 6-0 nylon.
   C. Individual simple or vertical mattress stitches are best for everting skin edges.

III. Cartilage repair
   A. If the cartilage is still attached to overlying skin and soft tissue, its blood supply should be intact. Care is taken when placing sutures through cartilage for fear of disrupting this blood supply.
   B. A large piece of avulsed cartilage that has intact perichondrium may be placed in the wound and soft tissue closed over it. Small pieces of cartilage may be removed without significant cosmetic impairment.
   C. Up to 2 cm of helical rim may be lost with primary closure repair.

Avulsion

Small parts of the ear may be avulsed with minimal cosmetic or functional impairment. Depending on which part of the auricle has been avulsed, the piece may be discarded or reapproximated.

I. Primary repair
  A. If a portion of the auricle is nearly avulsed but attached by a skin remnant, the skin remnant is evaluated to determine if blood flow is adequate. If it is, the avulsed piece of tissue can be reapproximated at the time of injury.
  B. If the avulsed segment is small and blood supply is poor, it can be removed and the remaining auricle reapproximated. Additional tissue may need to be removed to allow for good closure.
  C. If the lobule is avulsed, primary closure of the remaining soft tissue is performed. The lobule may be reconstructed at a later time.

II. Delayed repair
  Delayed repair is usually reserved for those cases in which a major portion of the auricle has been avulsed or when there is significant exposed cartilage without any viable skin.
  A. Remove the avulsed cartilage and adequately scrub it, removing all foreign debris.
  B. If debris is embedded in cartilage or soft tissue, dermabrasion is indicated.
  C. Primarily close the viable auricle that has an intact blood supply.
  D. Pocket principle
    1. If the avulsion occurs in association with numerous facial and head lacerations, a postauricular pocket can be created in one of the lacerations to store the avulsed piece of cartilage.
    2. An abdominal incision may also be used.
    3. Skin is removed from the avulsed segment.
    4. The cleansed, dermabraded, avulsed segment of cartilage is then buried within the pocket for 7 to 10 days. This allows for neovascularization and preserves good cartilage for grafting at a later date.

III. Postoperative care
  A. All patients are given antibiotics with coverage for *Staphylococcus aureus*.
  B. Antibiotic ointment may be placed over the suture lines.
  C. A mastoid dressing is applied for support. It should be firm enough to prevent mobility but not so tight as to impede blood flow. The dressing can be changed periodically for inspection of the wound. The dressing should stay in place 7 to 10 days in cases of avulsion. The dressing is removed immediately and the wound inspected if the patient complains of persistent pain, fever, or facial swelling.

Hematoma

Auricular hematomas are usually the result of blunt trauma to the ear (Fig. 1-1). They classically occur in boxers and can result in the cosmetic deformity known as a "cauliflower ear" (Fig. 1-2).[1]

I. Signs and symptoms
   A. Swelling
   B. Anterior displacement of the auricle
   C. A doughy consistency to the concha and the antihelix
   D. Pain
II. Treatment
   A. Aspiration of the hematoma is possible if performed immediately after the injury (Fig. 1-3).
   B. The hematoma is incised and drained (Fig. 1-3). The incision is made at the lateral aspect of the concha. This is generally necessary, as the clot is usually formed at the time of presentation.
   C. A Penrose drain is placed in the wound after evacuation of the clot.
   D. A mastoid pressure dressing is then placed and secured.
   E. Oral antibiotics with *Staphylococcus aureus* coverage are immediately instituted.
III. Complications

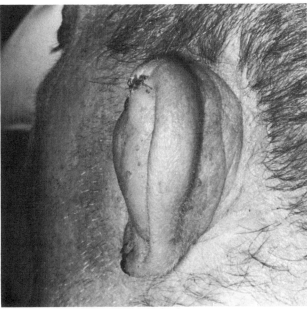

Fig. 1-1. Auricular hematoma.

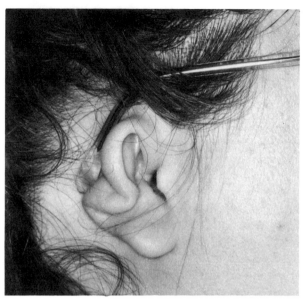

Fig. 1-2. Cauliflower ear.

A. Cauliflower ear. This occurs because of cartilage necrosis from enzymatic resorption and pressure changes from the hematoma secondarily interrupting the blood supply. A cauliflower ear not only produces significant cosmetic morbidity but may also cause functional impairment of hearing.

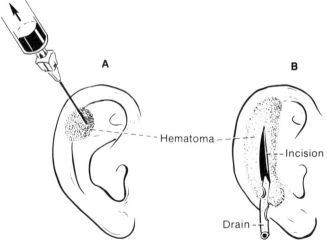

Fig. 1-3. (**A**) Aspiration of an early auricular hematoma. (**B**) Incision and drainage of an auricular hematoma.

B. Infection
C. Persistent pain

Abrasions

Most abrasions of the auricle cause significant pain and discomfort but little morbidity. Fortunately, they can be readily treated with adequate cleansing. Warm, sudsy water and gauze pads are usually the best form of cleansing. If grease is embedded in the abrasion, ether is used. If significant foreign body debris is present, it may be necessary to anesthetize the ear before beginning to scrub it. If the debris cannot be adequately removed by manual scrubbing, dermabrasion may be employed. Great care is taken to remove all foreign body debris, as leaving this behind will cause permanent tattooing.

Burns

The external ear is particularly vulnerable to thermal assault because of its exposed position and paucity of subcutaneous tissue. There are two ways that burns can damage the ear[2]: (1) Direct thermal injury may cause a full-thickness burn that results in autoamputation. (2) Secondary infection may follow a thermal injury.
  I. Treatment
    A. Avoid any pressure on the ear. Use a ring-shaped pillow to support the head when the patient lies down.
    B. Remember that the skin is nature's best dressing. If there is no immediate and obvious loss of cartilage, allow a dry eschar to form. This protects the ear from secretions coming from burned areas on the scalp.
    C. Allow separation of the eschar to progress naturally. Unless there is evidence of active infection underneath the eschar, the latter is left in place.
    D. If the tissue becomes necrotic, it can be débrided within 24 to 48 hours and a split-thickness skin graft placed.
    E. Apply mafenide acetate cream or sulfacetamide topically over the burned areas. This can be done in conjunction with dressings that are changed once or twice daily. These methods have been found to reduce surface contamination, and they maintain a softer texture of the burn eschar. With less edema forming, the vascularity is preserved and progressive necrosis can be avoided.
    F. Avoid systemic antibiotics unless infection is suspected.
    G. Débridement is not performed until necrotic tissue is evident. Excision can be delayed as long as 4 to 5 days after the thermal injury.
  II. Complications
    A. Infection

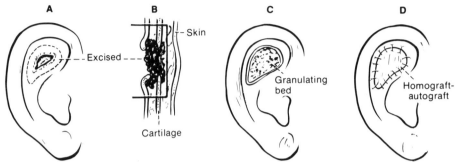

Fig. 1-4. Excision of necrotic skin and soft tissue in a case in chrondritis with secondary skin grafting. (**A**) Skin and cartilage to be excised. (**B**) Cross section of excised tissue. (**C**) Skin grafting is delayed until the infection has cleared and a granulating bed has developed. (**D**) Skin graft.

    B. Chondritis[3]
        1. Signs and symptoms
           a) Dull pain: the most prominent feature and increases in severity
           b) Erythema, warmth, fluctuance, and edema
           c) Tenderness
           d) Increase in the auriculocephalic angle
        2. Treatment
           a) Once chondritis has been documented, an incision and débridement of all necrotic tissue must be performed.
           b) At this point antibiotics may be instituted with coverage selected for *Staphylococcus aureus* and *Pseudomonas aeruginosa.*
           c) If an anesthetic is needed, 4 to 5 cc of lidocaine with 1:200,000 epinephrine may be injected in the posterior cartilaginous canal.
           d) A bivalve technique has been reported for auricular chondritis.
           e) Excision of the anterior wall of the abscess, including all necrotic cartilage and a thin rim of normal cartilage, is an alternative form of auricular preservation. Only the posterior skin remains as the base of the defect. A homograft skin graft is performed simultaneously (Fig. 1-4).
III. Secondary reconstruction
    A. Split-thickness skin graft. After the third postburn week, granulation tissue should be evident and a split-thickness skin graft can be easily performed. This is the most conservative form of treatment.
    B. Flap. A tubed pedicle flap has been used in the past when the helical rim is missing but is not a treatment of choice at this time. This technique requires a two-stage procedure and has no advantages over the other methods.
    C. Homograft cartilage, particularly the ninth or tenth costal cartilage, may be used in the auricular reconstruction.

Frostbite

The treatment and pathogenesis of frostbite is controversial. There are two schools of thought regarding the etiology of this condition: the first relates to tissue damage secondary to blood vessel injury, and the second relates to the direct action of the cold on the soft tissue providing a true thermal injury.[4]

I.   Classification
  A. First degree: edema and erythema of the skin
  B. Second degree: full demarcation
  C. Third degree: necrosis of the skin and subcutaneous tissues without autoamputation
  D. Fourth degree: necrosis with gangrene or autoamputation
II. Signs and symptoms
  A. Tissue pallor due to initial vasoconstriction and loss of circulation
  B. Formation of vesicles and bullae after tissue thaws
  C. Line of demarcation revealing erythema between the frozen and unfrozen tissue areas
  D. After 72 hours, frozen tissue reversion to normal or proceeding to necrosis
  E. Increased auriculocephalic angle
  F. Normal sensation until blebs appear and separate the epidermis from underlying tissue
  G. Alcohol intoxication sometimes a factor in the pathogenesis of frostbite
III. Good prognostic signs
  A. Warm ear
  B. Good color
  C. Large, clear blebs appearing early
  D. Persistence of skin sensation to pinprick
IV. Treatment
  A. Rapid rewarming with wet sterile cotton pledgets (108° to 110°F). Do not rewarm with ice, snow, or excessive heat. The use of extreme temperatures can have disastrous results.
  B. Sedatives and analgesics. Because the rewarming process can be quite painful the patient is sedated and kept as pain-free as possible.
  C. Maintain sterility, as this is an opportune time for infection. Systemic antibiotics are not used unless there is evidence of severe infection or sepsis.
  D. Silver nitrate soaks (0.5%) may be used for superficial infections.
  E. Do not débride the ear. The skin and bullae act as nature's best dressing and should be kept intact.
  F. No smoking. Because tobacco causes further vasoconstriction, a patient is restricted from smoking and from being around cigarette smokers.
V.   Long-term complications
  A. Hyperhidrosis

B. Severe sensitivity to extremes of cold and warm temperature
C. Neurovascular deficit—anesthesia or hyperesthesia

EXTERNAL AUDITORY CANAL

Foreign Bodies

See Chapter 13.

Lacerations

Lacerations may be caused by a variety of instruments including cotton-tipped applicators, hairpins, and sticks. They may also follow significant head and neck trauma. Because of the great vascularity of the external auditory canal, even a small laceration may result in copious bleeding. This usually stops spontaneously and is no excuse for avoiding a thorough examination.

I. Inspection
   A. Place the patient in a supine position.
   B. If a microscope is available, use it.
   C. Carefully suction with a 5 French suction tip.
   D. Take the time to ascertain where the injuries are. If there is a laceration of the anterior external auditory canal, the condyle of the mandible is inspected for a fracture. The condyle may be driven through the anterior wall of the cartilaginous external auditory canal causing a significant laceration.
   E. Check for an associated laceration of the tympanic membrane.
   F. Remove blood and debris with suction and cotton-tipped applicators.
   G. If the patient is complaining of significant pain, a postauricular block using 1% lidocaine with 1:100,000 epinephrine may be performed.
II. Repair
   A. Superficial lacerations of the external auditory canal need not be repaired, as they heal well.
   B. Circumferential lacerations are more ominous. They may result in canal stenosis. Antibiotic otic drops are instilled four times a day for 5 to 7 days, and long-term observation is warranted. If a stenosis seems to be forming, the antibiotic drops are continued and a wick is placed in the ear canal. An otolaryngologist is then consulted.
   C. Avulsion of significant amounts of soft tissue or skin may require a split-thickness skin graft. The best donor site is the postauricular area. After placement of the split-thickness skin graft a fingercot that has been filled with petroleum jelly-coated gauze may be placed as a stent.

Fractures

Fracture of the external auditory canal usually accompanies other temporal bone or mandibular fractures. If the anterior wall of the external auditory canal is fractured, the condyle of the mandible is inspected for a fracture. The two most common sites of external auditory canal fracture are the anterior canal and the tympanic ring.

I. Immediate treatment
   A. Carefully inspect the canal and remove any foreign body, debris, soft tissue, or extruded bone.
   B. Reduce the fracture. This may be performed by opening a nasal speculum in the ear canal after administering a local anesthetic.
   C. Position soft tissue or skin over the area of injury.
   D. Place the patient on an antibiotic otic suspension.
II. Delayed repair
   Delayed repair may be performed at the time of definitive reduction of other fractures.

Cerebrospinal Fluid Otorrhea

I. Evaluation
   Evaluation is performed carefully with as few instruments as possible. All instruments must be sterile.
   A. With the tympanic membrane intact, the eustachian tube is the conduit for the transfer of cerebrospinal fluid (CSF). With a small leak the amount of fluid arising in the nasopharynx is unnoticeable. With a large leak, however, the patient may be very conscious of fluid in the nasopharynx.
      1. Inspect the tympanic membrane for evidence of fluid in the middle ear. An air–fluid interface may present as a meniscus or air bubbles. Pneumatic otoscopy is not performed for fear of causing a pneumocephalus.
      2. Have the patient lean forward and note any significant rhinorrhea.
      3. Inspection of bloody rhinorrhea on a white cloth should reveal a ring sign, with the CSF having a further diffusion point than blood.
   B. If the tympanic membrane has been torn, the majority of CSF drains through the external auditory canal.
      1. Suction carefully and inspect with the aid of a microscope.
      2. Use the minimal amount of instrumentation that allows accurate diagnosis.
      3. Use only sterile instruments.
      4. Remove any foreign debris.
      5. Determine which quadrant of the tympanic membrane has been perforated.

6. After adequate inspection and diagnosis, place a sterile cotton ball in the external auditory canal. No further manipulation is performed; this includes pneumatic otoscopy.
7. Elevate the patient's head to a 30 degree angle.
8. Instruct the nurse to replace the cotton ball only as it becomes saturated.
9. Maintain bed rest while the patient has an obvious leak.
10. Most cases of CSF otorrhea resolve spontaneously within 72 hours. If there is no improvement after 2 weeks, surgical intervention is warranted.

II. Treatment
   A. Otic drops are contraindicated because they may contaminate the CSF with organisms from the external ear canal.
   B. Antibiotics are instituted only in cases of meningitis or sepsis. Oral antibiotics have no role.

TYMPANIC MEMBRANE, MIDDLE EAR, AND MASTOID

Traumatic Tympanic Membrane Perforation

I. Without associated injury and clean
   A. Most clean tympanic membrane perforations are caused by sharp instrumentation or a swift, blunt blow to the auricle.
   B. Most appear in the anterior-inferior quadrant of the pars tensa (Fig. 1-5).
   C. Antibiotics and otic drops are not indicated in a dry perforation.
   D. Ninety-five percent of these perforations heal spontaneously.
   E. Tuning forks classically illustrate a mild conductive component with the Weber localizing to the side of the injury (Figs. 1-6 and 1-7).

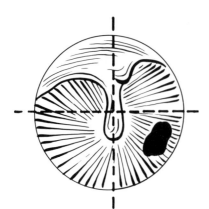

Fig. 1-5. Most traumatic tympanic membrane perforations occur in the anterior inferior quadrant.

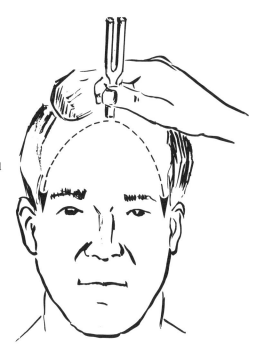

Fig. 1-6. Weber test with tuning fork placed on a bony midline structure.

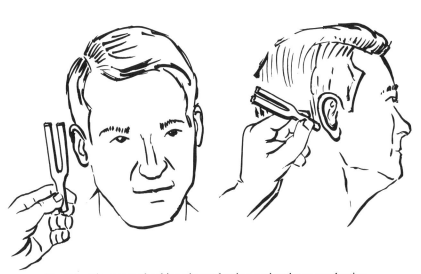

Fig. 1-7. Rinne test checking air conduction against bone conduction.

    F. In the patient who complains of decreased hearing a cigarette paper patch or a pressed Gelfoam patch may be placed over the tympanic membrane perforation. Tuning forks at that time should show restoration of hearing.

II. Contaminated injuries, usually following water accidents, e.g., water skiing. Slag injuries may occur in welders and people who work in steel mills.

    A. Examination of the ear is the same as above.

    B. Care is taken to remove any foreign debris.

    C. After thorough examination, the patient is started on antibiotic otic drops—and oral antibiotics if there is significant secondary infection.

    D. Healing is usually retarded in these patients. Particular care is paid to the patient with the molten slag injury. These ears may become severely infected after 1 to 2 weeks and may result in a severe tympanic membrane loss.

III. Site of injury

    A. More than 95% of all tympanic membrane perforations occur in the pars tensa.

    B. Care is taken to inspect the posterior-superior quadrant because of possible damage to the incudostapedial joint.

    C. Pars flaccida injuries usually result from sharp trauma.

Perforation with Ossicular Disruption[5]

I. Diagnosis

    A. The average anterior-inferior perforation does not have associated injury.

    B. Care is taken when evaluating the patient with a posterior-superior tympanic membrane perforation because of associated damage to the incudostapedial joint (Fig. 1-8). These patients have associated conductive and/or sensorineural hearing loss. *Note:* Pneumatic otoscopy should *not* be performed because of the risk of pneumocephalus.

    C. Tuning forks (256, 512, and 1,024 Hz) localize to the side of the injury.

    D. The maximum conductive hearing loss is 60 dB (average 45 dB).

II. Treatment

    A. The hearing mechanism need not be repaired immediately. A clean injury is allowed to heal with surgery planned at a later date. With a contaminated injury, antibiotic otic drops are administered and surgery scheduled when there is no threat of infection.

    B. Incudostapedial joint separation is the most common ossicular disruption. Often reconstruction requires only repositioning the lenticular process of the incus on the superstructure of the stapes. In more complicated

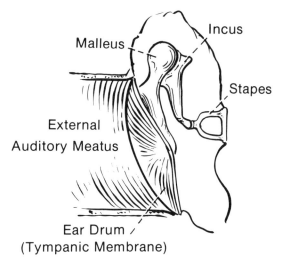

Fig. 1-8. Normal anatomy of the middle ear.

cases the incus may need to be removed and an incus interposition performed.

Injury with Associated Dizziness

Most injuries with dizziness involve injury to the posterior-superior quadrant of the tympanic membrane with subluxation of the incus on the stapes superstructure or displacement of the stapes into the vestibule.

I. Symptoms
   A. Nausea
   B. Vomiting
   C. Gait instability
   D. Nystagmus beating away from the injured side

II. Acute management
   The patient is placed in a comfortable position, sedated, and given anti-emetics as needed. Excellent drugs include droperidol or diazepam for sedation or promethazine hydrochloride suppositories 25 to 50 mg rectally q6h for nausea. The ear is then evaluated as previously described.

III. Complete evaluation
   A. Audiogram
   B. Temporal bone tomogram
   C. Electronystagmography (ENG): Avoid injecting water into the injured ear because of possible introduction of infection.

IV. Treatment
   Surgery is performed if a fistula between the inner ear and middle ear is suspected.

Injury with Complete Hearing Loss

I. Tuning forks (256, 512, and 1,024 Hz) localize to the noninjured side on the Weber test. The Rinne test reveals no hearing.
II. All patients with traumatically induced complete hearing loss are admitted to the hospital for evaluation:
    A. History and physical examination
    B. Audiogram
    C. Temporal bone tomograms
    D. Bed rest
    E. ENG without the caloric component
    F. Surgical exploration, if a fistula is suspected

INNER EAR
Temporal Bone Fracture

   See also Chapter 12.
I. Longitudinal temporal bone fracture (Fig. 1-9).
    A. Method of injury
       The direction of force in a longitudinal temporal bone fracture involves trauma to the parietal or temporal bone. The fracture extends

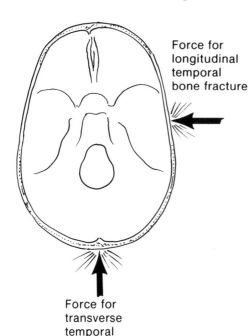

Force for longitudinal temporal bone fracture

Fig. 1-9. Direction of insult to produce transverse and longitudinal temporal bone fractures.

Force for transverse temporal bone fracture

from the external auditory canal anteromedially along the anterior edge of the petrous apex to the foramen lacerum and foramen ovale.

B. Hearing loss

1. Conductive hearing loss is present in a majority of cases.
2. Hemotympanum is common.
3. CSF may be found in the middle ear cavity.
4. Ossicular disruption is common.

C. Facial nerve

The facial nerve is injured in 20% of longitudinal temporal bone fractures. The site of injury is usually at the geniculate ganglion and horizontal (tympanic) portion of the facial nerve.

D. Associated injuries

1. Fracture of tympanic ring
2. Laceration of tympanic membrane
3. Ossicular discontinuity
4. Concussion

II. Transverse temporal bone fracture (Fig. 1-9)

A. Method of injury

The force is usually directed at the occiput. These fractures are extensions of posterior fossa fractures. The fracture line extends from the jugular foramen through the internal auditory canal to the foramen lacerum or foramen spinosum.

B. Hearing loss

1. A patient may be anacoustic with a fracture through the otic capsule.
2. Tuning forks localize to the good ear. The majority of patients have a mixed hearing loss with a large sensorineural component. Tuning forks may localize the site of injury, with air conduction being equal to bone conduction.

C. Facial nerve

Fifty percent of transverse temporal bone fractures are associated with facial nerve injury. The most common site of involvement is just distal to the otic capsule.

D. Associated injuries

1. Other skull fractures
2. Concussions

Inner Ear Concussion

I. Sensorineural hearing loss

The injury may be due to a fracture through the otic capsule or to concussive damage to the cochlea.

A. Obtain a thorough history as to the type of trauma sustained and the direction of force.

B. Perform a thorough otologic and cranial nerve examination.

   C. Tuning forks classically reveal a sensorineural hearing loss. The Weber test lateralizes to the side opposite the injury, and air conduction is greater than bone conduction on the side of the injury.

   D. Evaluation

      1. Audiogram

      2. ENG

      3. Temporal bone tomograms

      4. Computed tomography (CT scan)

   E. Prognosis

      A sensorineural hearing loss involving primarily the upper frequencies may have a good prognosis. With most hearing loss confined to the low frequencies, the prognosis is poor. The patient is observed and has several audiograms performed during the next 3 to 5 days. If there is stabilization of the hearing, audiograms are repeated in 1 to 2 weeks.

II. Dizziness

   A. Signs and symptoms

      1. Nausea

      2. Vomiting

      3. Gait instability

      4. Nystagmus away from injured side

   B. Site of lesion: located by ENG

   C. Immediate treatment

      1. Bed rest

      2. Diazepam 5 to 10 mg i.m. q6h or promethazine hydrochloride suppositories 25 to 50 mg per rectum q6h. Patients receiving these medications require close respiratory and cardiac monitoring.

      3. After vertigo has subsided, a formal evaluation with audiogram, ENG, and CT scan is performed.

REFERENCES

1. English GM: Common injuries to the ear. Primary Care 3:507, 1976
2. Grant DA, Finley ML, Coers CR: Early management of the burned ear. Plast Reconstr Surg 44:161, 1969
3. Dowling JA, Foley FD, Moncrief JA: Chondritis in the burned ear. Plast Reconstr Surg 42:115, 1968
4. Sessions DG, Stallings JO, Mills W, Beal D: Frostbite of the ear. Laryngoscope 80:1223, 1970
5. Myers D, Schlosser W, Wolfson RJ, et al: Otologic diagnosis and the treatment of deafness. Clin Symp, 1962

2

Trauma to the Face and Scalp

Stephen J. Wetmore

Although some scalp injuries result in significant blood loss, most face and scalp soft tissue injuries and most facial bone fractures do not result in immediate life-threatening situations. When a patient with multiple injuries is seen in the emergency room, a cursory examination of the scalp and face usually reveals evidence of life-threatening problems such as major hemorrhage or airway obstruction. If such problems are not evident, the examiner checks for other life-threatening injuries, e.g., epidural or subdural hemorrhage, cervical spine injury, laryngotracheal injury, tension pneumothorax, or ruptured spleen, before performing a thorough examination of the face and scalp. Documentation of facial injuries by drawings and photographs is usually worthwhile prior to repair of the injuries.

FACIAL AND SCALP SOFT TISSUE INJURIES

Lacerations

I. Control of hemorrhage
   A. Pressure applied directly to the bleeding site controls most facial and scalp hemorrhage at least temporarily.
   B. A hemostat is applied to large vessels that continue to bleed after direct pressure is removed. Chromic or silk suture can be used to ligate these vessels.
   C. Scalp lacerations that bleed profusely from many vessels can be controlled by using a 2-0 nylon running suture taking large, deep bites.
II. Evaluation of injury
   A. Scalp: check for skull fracture or foreign body.
   B. Face: check for facial nerve injuries and underlying bone injuries.
III. Repair of lacerations[1,2]
   A. Anesthesia
      1. Local anesthesia
         a) Check for facial nerve injury prior to injecting the local anesthetic agent.

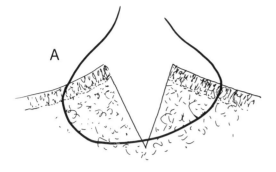

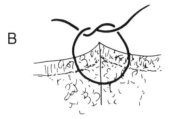

Fig. 2-1. (**A**) The needle is inserted further laterally in the subdermal tissue, then in the epidermis. (**B**) The skin edges are thereby everted, which produces a better scar.

       b) Use 1% lidocaine with 1:100,000 epinephrine; if the tissues' blood supply appears to be compromised use lidocaine without epinephrine.

       c) Sedation is usually unnecessary after local block.

    2. General anesthesia

       a) Usually needed for major wounds

       b) Occasionally needed in an uncooperative patient

B. Cleansing and débridement

    1. Dirt and other foreign substances removed with soap scrub

    2. Copious irrigation with saline

    3. Excision of nonviable tissues

    4. Avoid extensive débridement; the face and scalp have an excellent blood supply and most tissues survive unless they are obviously nonviable.

C. Primary closure of lacerations

    1. Sew in layers if deep laceration.

    2. Avoid tension on skin edges.

    3. Evert skin edges by taking larger bites of subdermal tissue than of epidermis (Fig. 2-1).

    4. Suture selection

       a) Chromic 3-0 or 4-0 to close deep layers of face, 2-0 or 3-0 chromic for deep scalp.

       b) Nylon or prolene 5-0 or 6-0 for skin of face.

       c) Nylon or prolene 3-0 or 4-0 for scalp.

    5. Steri-strips

a) Useful in small or superficial lacerations, especially in children
   b) Also useful in splinting lacerations after early removal of skin sutures
6. Specific lacerations
   a) Lip. First line up vermilion border (mucocutaneous junction) carefully. Then place deep sutures if necessary.
   b) Nasal ala. Evert edges carefully to try to avoid notch deformity from scar contracture.
   c) Intraoral degloving injury (an injury in which the mucosa is sheared from the mandible or maxilla at the junction of the firmly attached gum mucosa and the loosely attached lip mucosa). Suture with absorbable material. Sew around teeth if necessary.
   d) Tongue. Slowly absorbable suture such as Dexon or Vicryl is considered if a gaping injury is present; small laceration may be sutured with absorbable 3-0 or 4-0 chromic; unless the laceration is grossly contaminated, the mucosal laceration can be closed completely without drains.
7. Most lacerations of the face or scalp less than 24 hours old can be closed primarily with little risk of infection if they are fairly clean. Even lacerations that are open for more than 24 hours may be sutured primarily if they are clean.
D. Dressings
   1. Immobilization—usually unnecessary
   2. Pressure for hemostasis if indicated
E. Antibiotics
   1. Use empirically for deep or ''dirty'' lacerations.
   2. Penicillin covers most potential pathogens.
F. Tetanus prophylaxis[3]
   1. In previously immunized patient
      a) For clean minor wound, give toxoid 0.5 ml if more than 10 years has elapsed since last booster.
      b) For clean major wound or tetanus-prone wound, give toxoid 0.5 ml if at least 5 years has elapsed since last booster; if more than 10 years has elapsed, also give 250 units human tetanus immune globulin at another injection site.
   2. In patient who is not immunized or who is partially immunized
      a) For clean minor wound, give 0.5 ml toxoid and later complete the immunization schedule.
      b) For clean major or tetanus-prone wound, give human tetanus immune globulin 250 units in one arm and toxoid 0.5 ml in the other arm; later complete the tetanus immunization.
G. Removal of sutures
   1. Remove skin sutures in the face in 3 to 5 days. Remove sutures earlier in women or children and later in men.
   2. Scalp sutures should remain in place for about 7 days.

3. If wound closed under tension or if patient has severe metabolic problems, leave sutures in place a few days longer, or sutures can be removed at 3 to 5 days and Steri-strips used for another few days.

H. Scar maturation
   1. Raised red line for weeks to months
   2. Eventual white line scar
   3. Revision of scars not earlier than 6 months postinjury

Abrasions

I. Cleansing and débridement
   A. May need local anesthesia
   B. Gentle scrubbing
   C. Copious irrigation
   D. Débridement of nonviable tissue
II. Dressing
   A. Keep moist with antibiotic ointment.
   B. Occlusive dressings are avoided because wound may become infected.

Avulsions

I. Cleansing and débridement
II. Anesthesia
   Be careful of blood supply with near-avulsions. Use regional block in these cases.
III. Repair of injury
   A. Primary closure: If wound is small, the local tissues can be undermined and the wound closed primarily.
   B. Local flaps can be used if the physician is knowledgeable about them.
   C. Skin grafts
      1. Postauricular area: best color match
      2. Infraclavicular or supraclavicular area: good color match
      3. Abdomen or thigh area: worst color match
   D. Healing by secondary intention
      1. Wound contraction is an active process by which the wound shrinks by "drawing in" surrounding normal skin.
      2. May be able to avoid using flaps or skin grafts.
      3. Disadvantages: It takes several weeks for complete healing, and there is the possibility of contractures that can distort the anatomy of the face.

Periorbital Trauma (Contusion or Black Eye)

I. Suspect a periorbital bone fracture.
   A. Nose
   B. Orbital rim
   C. Orbital floor
II. Examine for eye injury: vision, extraocular muscles, hyphema (hemorrhage in anterior chamber).
III. Treat the contusion.
   A. Cold compresses
   B. Elevation of head

FACIAL BONE FRACTURES

Nasal Fracture

See Fig. 2-2.
I. Introduction
   A. Most common type of facial fracture
   B. Usually due to direct trauma

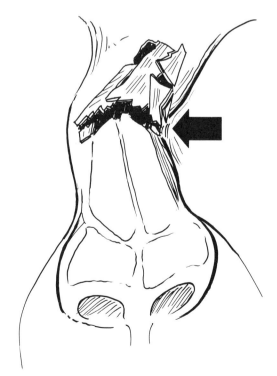

Fig. 2-2. The force of the blow fractures and deforms the nose.

    C. If nasal deformity present, ascertain if deformity was present prior to current trauma

II. Diagnosis
    A. Signs and symptoms
        1. Pain, tenderness, and swelling
        2. Epistaxis: almost always present but rarely severe
        3. External nasal deformity
        4. Internal nasal swelling
           a) Use a nasal speculum and a headlight.
           b) Inspect with use of topical anesthetics and decongestants.
        5. Septal hematoma
           a) Swelling of septum, usually bilateral
           b) Nasal obstruction
           c) If untreated, may result in infection and necrosis of septal cartilage with resultant saddle nose deformity
    B. X-ray examination
        Films are not necessary for isolated nasal fracture, as treatment depends on degree of external and internal deformity, which is usually quite evident on physical examination.

III. Treatment
    A. If markedly swollen, delay therapy for several days until swelling subsides.
        1. Ice packs
        2. Head elevation
        3. Antibiotics: penicillin effective against most potential pathogens
    B. Reduction of fracture
        1. Local anesthesia in most instances
           a) Cocaine spray or pledgets for topical use
           b) Lidocaine 1% with 1:100,000 epinephrine for injection
           c) May need narcotics intravenously or intramuscularly
        2. General anesthesia
           a) Child
           b) Uncooperative adult
        3. Instruments
           a) Asch forceps to straighten entire dorsum
           b) Freer or Ballenger elevator to push out depressed lateral nasal wall
        4. Dressings
           a) Gauze packing in nose
              (1) Commercially available 0.5 inch Vaseline gauze, *or*
              (2) Add antibiotic ointment to 0.5 inch plain gauze
           b) Splint over dorsum
              (1) Tape
              (2) Plaster cast or prefabricated splint
    C. Septal hematoma

        1. Incise and drain
        2. Gauze packing
        3. Antibiotics
    D. Nondisplaced fracture
       Avoid contact sports for 6 weeks.

Mandible Fracture

I. Introduction
    A. Motor vehicle accidents and altercations are common causes.
    B. Check for associated injuries, especially a cervical spine fracture.
        1. If patient is unconscious, obtain lateral cervical spine films before extensive movement of patient.
        2. Airway compromise and hemorrhage may occur with severe mandible fractures.
II. Diagnosis
    A. Signs and symptoms
        1. Pain, swelling, localized tenderness, and trismus
        2. Malocclusion
        3. Gingival mucosal tears
    B. Look for more than one mandible fracture.
    C. May have associated midface injuries.
    D. X-ray examination
        1. Panoramic x-ray film of mandible
        2. Plain films of mandible if panoramic x-ray film not available
III. Treatment
    A. Airway distress and/or severe bleeding
        1. Unusual from isolated mandible fracture but can occur with severely displaced fractures.
        2. Endotracheal intubation may be difficult, and tracheotomy may be necessary.
        3. Consider possibility of laryngotracheal separation from blunt trauma to neck.
    B. Displaced mandible fractures with intraoral gingival tear
        1. Immediate treatment
           a) Antibiotics: penicillin
           b) May undergo immediate repair in operating room, or repair may be delayed for several days.
           c) If external lacerations are present, immediate repair of fracture and closure of lacerations are indicated.
        2. Delayed repair
           a) If repair is delayed, patient may be placed on liquid diet.

     b) Delay may be necessary in order to provide time to manufacture surgical splints or to ensure that other injuries do not jeopardize patient's life.

     c) If marked displacement is present, consider temporary wiring together of the two teeth adjacent to the fracture to splint the fracture and increase patient comfort.

C. Mandible fracture without mucosal tears or with minimal displacement and without associated injuries

  1. Usually needs surgical therapy but may have operation performed within 7 to 10 days after injury without undue jeopardy

  2. Often does not need emergency hospitalization but can be temporarily sent home on soft diet with instructions to return for elective admission for surgery

D. Types of surgical therapy

  1. Depends on severity of fracture(s), location of fracture(s), status of teeth, and presence of associated facial and other injuries

  2. Intermaxillary (between maxilla and mandible) fixation[4]

     a) Wires are used to position an arch bar on both the mandibular and maxillary teeth, and then the teeth are fixed together in occlusion by attaching wires or rubber bands between the arch bars (Fig. 2-3).

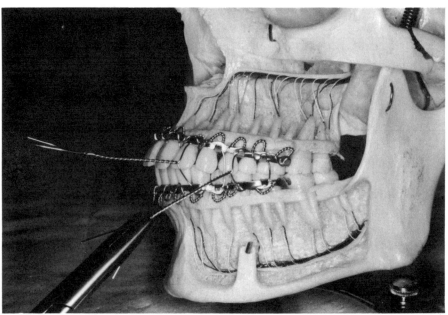

Fig. 2-3. Intermaxillary fixation wires are placed between the maxillary and mandibular arch bars to immobilize the fracture(s).

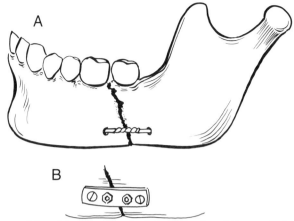

Fig. 2-4. (A) Direct wiring of fracture near the inferior border of the mandible. (B) A bone plate is an alternative method for reduction and fixation of a mandible fracture.

    b) Six weeks of fixation is usually necessary in adults and 4 weeks in children.
  3. Open reduction and internal fixation
    a) Either extraoral or intraoral approach with reduction and direct wiring of the bone fragments (Fig. 2-4)
    b) Usually requires intermaxillary fixation for 6 weeks
  4. Surgical splints[5]

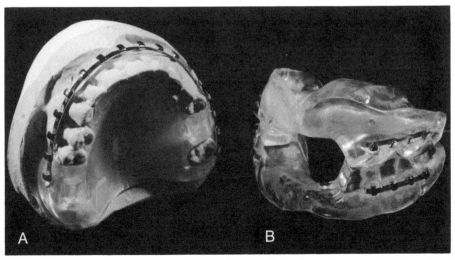

Fig. 2-5. (A) The palatal splint compensates for the multiple missing molar teeth. (B) The modified Gunning splint is used in edentulous patients.

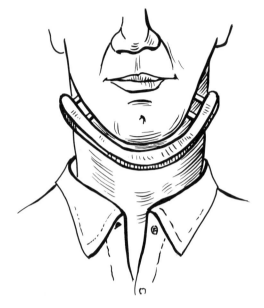

Fig. 2-6. The biphase technique consists of external fixation by an acrylic bar that is attached to screws which are placed into the mandible.

    a) Frequently used for edentulous patients but may also be useful in children with deciduous teeth, in adults with multiple missing teeth, and for severely comminuted fractures

    b) Fashioned from acrylic (Fig. 2-5) or from patient's own dentures

  5. Other forms of surgical therapy

    a) Biphase external fixation devices (Fig. 2-6). Intermaxillary fixation may often be omitted with this technique.

    b) Bone plates (Fig. 2-4)

  6. Certain selected mandible fractures may be successfully treated with soft diet and without surgical intervention.

Midface Fractures

Maxillary Bone Fractures (Le Fort Fractures)[4]

  I. Introduction

    A. Less common than nasal or mandible fractures

    B. Often associated with motor vehicle accidents

  II. Diagnosis

    A. Signs and symptoms

      1. Pain, tenderness, swelling of midface

      2. Malocclusion

      3. "Floating" maxilla

      4. Nosebleed and nasal obstruction

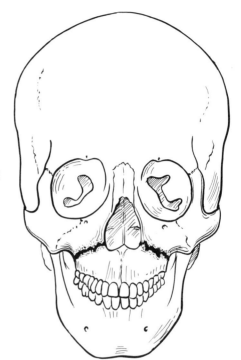

Fig. 2-7. LeFort I. The fracture line is located just above the hard palate.

5. Often associated with nasal or mandible fractures
6. Possible periorbital swelling, ecchymosis, scleral hemorrhage, and eye injury

B. X-ray examination
  1. Waters and lateral views are most helpful in determining the extent of the fracture.
  2. Fracture lines and air–fluid levels (blood) or mucosal thickening or opacity are often present in the maxillary sinuses.
  3. Tomograms or computed tomography (CT scan) are useful in extensive injuries.

C. LeFort classification
  1. LeFort I—separates hard palate from rest of maxilla (Fig. 2-7).
  2. LeFort II—pyramidal fracture to orbital rims (Fig. 2-8)
  3. LeFort III—midface separation from skull
  4. Often a combination of fractures are present (Fig. 2-9).

III. Therapy
  A. Treat associated injuries.
  B. Antibiotics—prophylactic
    1. Nasal mucosa usually torn
    2. Blood in maxillary sinuses

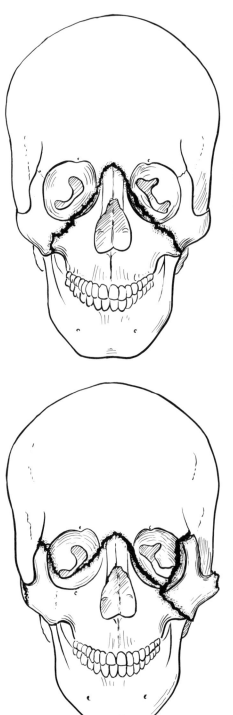

Fig. 2-8. LeFort II. This pyramidal type of fracture extends across the inferior orbital rim and continues superiorly to cross the dorsum of the nose.

Fig. 2-9. A LeFort III fracture is present on the right side, and a LeFort II fracture and a tripod fracture are present on the left side.

    C. Avoid blowing nose because it may result in subcutaneous emphysema.

    D. Surgical therapy is usually necessary.

       1. Reduce fractures and place in intermaxillary fixation.

       2. Suspend fractured maxilla from stable points on the skull.

       3. Temporary tracheotomy may be necessary because nasal swelling may prevent adequate breathing while teeth are wired together during the immediate postoperative period.

    E. Teeth are usually kept in occlusion for at least 6 weeks.

Tripod Fracture (Trimalar Fracture, Zygomaticomaxillary Fracture)

  See Figs. 2-9, and 2-10.

  I. Introduction

    A. Commonly seen after motor vehicle accident or altercation

    B. May be seen in conjunction with maxillary fracture

    C. Characteristically has three fracture lines

       1. Frontozygomatic suture line

       2. Zygomatic arch

       3. Orbital rim—extends from infraorbital nerve foramen inferiorly over the face of the maxilla

  II. Diagnosis

    A. Signs and symptoms

       1. Swelling over malar eminence

       2. Subconjunctival hemorrhage

       3. Localized tenderness over fracture lines

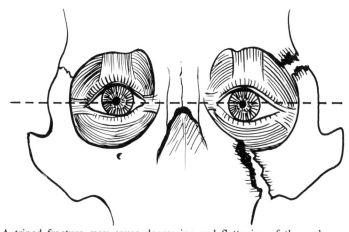

Fig. 2-10. A tripod fracture may cause depression and flattening of the malar eminence and enophthalmos.

4. Flattening of malar eminence—usually occurs if the fracture is displaced, but may be disguised for first few days after injury by swelling
5. Trismus—possible if coronoid process is trapped by a depressed segment of the zygomatic arch
6. Periorbital swelling and ecchymosis
7. Anesthesia over cheek in distribution of infraorbital nerve
8. Possible eye (globe) injury
9. Possible limitation of motion in upward gaze from inferior rectus muscle entrapment, edema, or oculomotor nerve injury
10. Forced duction test can differentiate muscle entrapment from oculomotor nerve injury; after anesthetizing the conjunctiva, the inferior rectus muscle is grasped with an iris forcep and the mobility of the globe determined. If the inferior rectus is entrapped, upward movement is limited. If upward mobility is unimpaired by forced duction, an oculomotor nerve injury is presumed.

B. X-ray examination
1. Waters view is the most helpful view.
2. Look for the three main fractures listed above as well as for mucosal thickening, air–fluid levels, or opacity of the maxillary sinus.
3. Look also for a soft tissue shadow projecting from the floor of the orbit into the maxillary sinus, as herniation of orbital contents into the sinus can occur.
4. Tomograms or CT scans may be helpful to better delineate orbital floor injuries and are useful in severe injuries to delineate the extent of injury.

C. Ophthalmology consultation to diagnose and treat possible intraocular injury

III. Treatment
A. Ice packs and elevation of head
B. Surgical therapy
1. Multiple approaches depending on the extent of injury
2. Brow incision to reduce fracture and wire frontozygomatic suture separation
3. Lower lid incision to reduce and wire the orbital rim component
4. Orbital floor exploration through a lower lid incision, perhaps, to relieve entrapment of the inferior rectus or to reduce a large depressed orbital floor fracture
5. Maxillary sinus antrotomy (Caldwell-Luc approach) if orbital floor requires packing in order to hold it into proper alignment

Orbital Floor (Blowout) Fracture

See Fig. 2-11.
I. Introduction
A. Differentiated from tripod fracture in that the orbital rim is intact

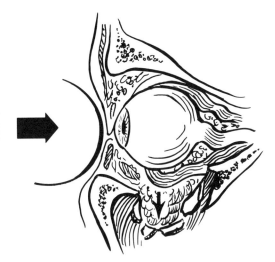

Fig. 2-11. An orbital floor (blowout) fracture results from a direct force applied to the eye with fracture of the thin bone of the orbital floor.

B. Often due to a ball or a fist hitting the eye
C. Mechanism of injury is a sudden increase of intraorbital pressure causing a fracture of the thin orbital floor resulting in partial prolapse of orbital contents into the maxillary sinus
D. Higher incidence of globe injury than in tripod fracture

II. Diagnosis
   A. Signs and symptoms
      1. Periorbital swelling and ecchymosis
      2. Subconjunctival hemorrhage
      3. Sometimes proptosis initially
      4. Enophthalmos (eye sunken in and down in orbit), possible late sequela
      5. Diplopia, often, possibly due to entrapment of inferior rectus muscle at fracture site, edema of orbit, or oculomotor nerve injury
      6. Forced duction test to differentiate muscle entrapment from nerve injury. See tripod fracture diagnosis.
   B. X-ray examination
      1. Waters and lateral views are most helpful to look for defects of the orbital floor and herniation of orbital contents into the maxillary sinus.
      2. Tomograms or CT scans often are helpful to delineate the exact location of the orbital floor defect.
   C. Ophthalmology consultation
      Blowout fractures are associated with a higher incidence of ocular injuries than are tripod fractures.[6]

III. Treatment
   Surgical treatment is controversial.

A. If entrapment of the inferior rectus is present or if a large amount of orbital tissue has dropped into the maxillary sinus, orbital floor repair is indicated.

B. If diplopia and enophthalmos is absent and the amount of orbital contents herniated into the maxillary sinus is minimal, immediate surgical intervention is probably not necessary.

C. Delayed orbital floor exploration with insertion of an orbital floor implant may be necessary if enophthalmos and/or diplopia occur as late sequelae of an untreated fracture.

D. Occasionally orbital fat necrosis occurs either in a treated or untreated fracture with resultant enophthalmos. An orbital implant may be necessary to raise the level of the globe.

Depressed Zygomatic Arch Fracture

See Fig. 2-12.
I. Introduction
   A. Zygomatic arch fracture is one of the components of a tripod fracture, but an isolated zygomatic arch fracture may result from a direct blow to the arch.
   B. Nondisplaced fractures require no treatment, but most comminuted depressed zygomatic arch fractures should be treated.
II. Diagnosis
   A. Signs and symptoms
      1. Palpable depression localized to one portion of the zygomatic arch
      2. Pain, tenderness, and swelling over the fracture site

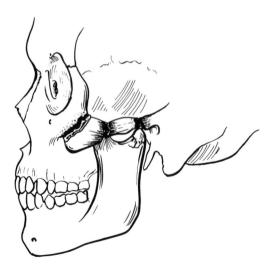

Fig. 2-12. The depressed fragments of the zygomatic arch fracture may impinge on the coronoid process of the mandible.

    3. Difficulty and pain upon opening and closing the jaw due to impingement of the fractured zygomatic arch on the coronoid process of the mandible

 B. X-ray examination

   Submental-vertex view of the face to demonstrate the depressed fragments

 C. Treatment

    1. Depressed zygomatic arch fractures usually require reduction.

    2. Gilles approach (incision in hairline of temporal region) or intraoral approach is used.

    3. Fractured segments may "pop" into place or may require stabilization with packing or extracranial traction.

Frontal Bone Fractures[7]

Nasofrontal (Nasoethmoid) Fracture

 I. Introduction

   Nasofrontal fracture is usually due to a direct blow to the nose with telescoping of the nasal bones and the inferior edge of the frontal bone into the ethmoid sinus region.

 II. Diagnosis

 A. Signs and symptoms

    1. Nasal deformity with depressed roof of nose, swelling, pain, and tenderness

    2. Epistaxis, rarely severe

    3. Periorbital ecchymosis and swelling, bilateral

    4. Subconjunctival hemorrhage, bilateral

    5. Telecanthus possible from injury to medial canthal ligament

    6. Cerebrospinal fluid (CSF) rhinorrhea, often seen with a fracture of the cribriform plate

 B. X-ray examination

    1. Sinus films

    2. Tomograms: often helpful to assess extent of fractures and to look for cribriform plate injury

 C. Ophthalmology consultation—high incidence of concomitant ocular injuries

 III. Treatment—surgical

 A. Closed reduction of nasal fracture with packing of nose to hold fragments into place may be all that is necessary in some patients.

 B. Open reduction of nasofrontal fracture may be necessary if medial canthal injury has occurred, if the anterior wall of frontal sinus is depressed, or if the nasofrontal ducts appear compromised.

C. If nasofrontal ducts are severely compromised (and they frequently are), obliteration of the frontal sinus with abdominal fat may be necessary.

D. If the frontal sinuses are not surgically obliterated, frontal sinus x-ray films are obtained a few months after injury to ensure that the frontal sinuses are reaerated.

E. If CSF leak persists after reduction of fractures, a craniotomy may be necessary to repair the dural defect which is usually in the region of the cribriform plates.

Frontal Sinus Fractures

See Fig. 2-13.

I. Introduction

Frontal sinus fracture is usually due to direct trauma to the forehead. A nondisplaced linear fracture of the anterior table usually does not require treatment, but a depressed anterior table fracture requires treatment to correct the cosmetic deformity that will result. Fractures through the nasofrontal ducts or posterior table of the frontal sinus may require surgical therapy to prevent mucocele or pyocele development or to repair a dural tear.

II. Diagnosis

A. Signs and symptoms

1. Pain, tenderness, swelling over the fracture site or on the forehead
2. Palpable depressed fracture possible
3. Lacerations at the fracture site frequently present
4. Periorbital ecchymosis and edema frequently present bilaterally

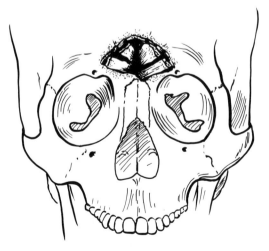

Fig. 2-13. Depressed fracture of the anterior table of the frontal sinus.

B. X-ray examination

   Sinus films may show the fracture, but tomograms or CT scans are useful to assess the extent of bone and soft tissue injury.

III. Treatment

   A. Lacerations are repaired.
   B. Isolated nondisplaced linear fracture of anterior table usually requires no surgical treatment.
   C. Depressed fracture of anterior table, fractures through the nasofrontal ducts, and posterior wall fractures usually require surgical therapy.

REFERENCES

1. Holt GR: Management of soft-tissue trauma. Ear Nose Throat J 62:393, 1983
2. Farrior RT, Jarchow RC, Rojas B: Primary and late plastic repair of soft tissue injuries. Otolaryngol Clin North Am 16:697, 1983
3. Walt AJ (ed): Early Care of the Injured Patient. p. 70. WB Saunders, Philadelphia, 1982
4. Dingman RO, Natvig P: Surgery of Facial Fractures. WB Saunders, Philadelphia, 1964
5. Jackson MJ, Wetmore SJ: Surgical prosthetic splints as an adjunct in treating facial fractures. Arch Otolaryngol 106:25, 1980
6. Crumley RL, Leibsohn J, Krause CJ, Burton TC: Fractures of the orbital floor. Laryngoscope 87:934, 1977
7. Holt GR: Ethmoid and frontal sinus fractures. Ear Nose Throat J 62:357, 1983

3

Trauma to the Neck

James Y. Suen

LARYNX AND TRACHEA

I. Introduction
   A. Significance
      1. Life-threatening
      2. Permanent airway problems
      3. Permanent voice changes
   B. Etiology
      1. Auto accidents—injuries from steering wheel or dashboard
      2. Stretched wires
      3. Hanging
      4. Gunshot wounds
      5. Other blunt objects, e.g., fist or foot
   C. General considerations
      1. Associated neck injuries, e.g., cervical spine fractures or vascular injuries
      2. Can occur with blunt trauma without skin lacerations or from penetrating injuries
      3. History and physical examination important: includes indirect mirror examination of larynx if no airway distress
II. Differential diagnosis (Fig. 3-1)
   A. Contusion
   B. Dislocation of the cricoarytenoid joint
   C. Fracture of the hyoid bone
   D. Fracture of the thyroid and/or cricoid cartilages
   E. Laryngotracheal separation; usually also recurrent laryngeal nerve injuries
III. Clinical manifestations
   A. Contusion
      1. Symptoms
         a) Pain
         b) Hoarseness
      2. Signs
         a) Tenderness of thyroid cartilages
         b) Edema
         c) Possible hematoma of the endolarynx
   B. Dislocated cricoarytenoid joint

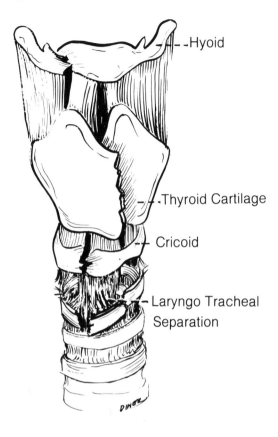
Hyoid

Thyroid Cartilage

Cricoid

Laryngo Tracheal
Separation

Fig. 3-1. Injuries that can occur with trauma to the larynx and trachea.

1. Symptoms
    a) Pain
    b) Hoarseness
    c) Mild dyspnea
    d) Dysphagia
    e) Slight aspiration
2. Signs
    a) Edema of the arytenoid area and aryepiglottic fold
    b) Abnormal arytenoid position
    c) Bowing and decreased mobility of vocal cord
C. Fractured hyoid bone
    1. Symptoms
        a) Pain
        b) Odynophagia
    2. Signs
        a) Tenderness and swelling over hyoid
        b) Bony crepitus

        c) Supraglottic edema

        d) Hematoma

  D. Fractured thyroid and/or cricoid cartilages

    1. Symptoms

        a) Pain

        b) Mild to severe dyspnea

        c) Stridor

        d) Hoarseness or aphonia

        c) Odynophagia

        f) Hemoptysis

    2. External neck signs

        a) Subcutaneous emphysema

        b) Loss of landmarks of external larynx

        c) Tenderness of larynx

        d) Palpable fracture of thyroid cartilage

        e) Ecchymosis of skin

    3. Internal neck examination

        a) Endolaryngeal edema or hematoma

        b) Distortion of normal anatomy

        c) Mucosal tears of larynx or posterior pharynx

        d) Bleeding

        e) Exposed cartilage

        f) Vocal cord weakness or displacement

  E. Laryngotracheal separation

    1. Symptoms

        a) Severe dyspnea

        b) Pain

        c) Aphonia or hoarseness

        d) Hemoptysis

        e) Odynophagia

    2. Signs

        a) Airway distress

        b) Subcutaneous emphysema

        c) Tenderness

        d) Swelling

        e) Ecchymosis

        f) Head posturing forward to breathe

        g) Laryngeal edema

        h) Paralyzed vocal cord

IV. Diagnostic studies

  A. Soft tissue radiographs of cervical area: anteroposterior (AP) and lateral views to examine the cervical spine, check for soft tissue free air, and check for laryngeal fractures

B. Chest x-ray film to check for mediastinal emphysema and/or pneumothorax
C. Laryngogram (seldom needed)—if no airway distress; may be obtained to check for mucosal tears
D. Computed tomography (CT scan)—if no airway distress; may be help-ful to localize fracture sites
E. Direct laryngoscopy—usually under general anesthesia to accurately assess the extent of injury; if major injury, performed at time of tra-cheotomy and corrective surgery

V. Treatment

With severe injuries to the larynx and trachea, airway obstruction is usually seen. It is very important to diagnose these injuries early and administer the appropriate treatment quickly.[1]

A. Immediate treatment
    1. Intubation: can be attempted if patient is semiconscious or uncon-scious. Intubation may be difficult because of the distorted larynx and trachea. Tracheotomy is preferred if subcutaneous emphysema is present.
    2. Tracheotomy or cricothyroidotomy
        a) Procedure of choice if patient is alert and having severe airway distress
        b) Usually is performed in sitting or semisitting position
        c) If person performing the tracheotomy is inexperienced, a cricothyroidotomy[2,3] is safer and quicker. It can be converted to a tracheotomy in 24 to 48 hours on an elective basis.
B. Intermediate treatment
    1. Contusion: If no airway distress or fracture, only voice rest, head elevation, and continued observation are necessary.
    2. Cricoarytenoid joint dislocation: Attempt relocation under general anesthesia with direct laryngoscopy within 48 hours.
    3. Fracture of the hyoid bone: Give symptomatic treatment or, rarely, open reduction and interosseous wiring of major fracture.
    4. Fracture of the thyroid and/or cricoid cartilage
        a) Tracheotomy
        b) Open reduction
        c) Stabilization
        d) Repair lacerations
        e) Insert stent
    5. Laryngotracheal separation
        a) Tracheotomy
        b) Open reduction
        c) Suture cartilages and insert stent.
        d) Explore recurrent laryngeal nerves.
        e) Consider reanastomosis of nerve if severed.

C. Ancillary treatment
  1. Administer antibiotics to try to prevent infections from mucosal tears and subcutaneous emphysema and to help avoid stenosis.
  2. Steroids are used for severe edema of larynx.

CERVICAL SPINE

I. Introduction
  A. Significance: If the cervical spine is fractured or dislocated, the condition may be life-threatening from neurogenic shock, or it may cause quadriplegia.
  B. Etiology
    1. Moving vehicle accidents
    2. Stretched wires
    3. Hanging
    4. Falls
    5. Swimming or water sports
  C. General considerations
    1. Associated injuries such as fractured larynx or vascular injuries
    2. May be in spinal shock
    3. Airway distress (must be managed first with neck immobilized)
II. Diagnosis
  A. Symptoms
    1. Neck pain
    2. Dyspnea
  B. Signs
    1. Neck swelling
    2. Tenderness over cervical vertebrae
    3. No neurologic abnormalities
    4. Paraplegia or quadriplegia
    5. Dyspnea
  C. Radiographic studies: AP and lateral views of cervical spine with arms and shoulders pulled caudally. (All cervical vertebrae should be visualized.) Look for dislocation of vertebrae and/or increased thickness of retropharyngeal space.
III. Differential diagnosis
  A. Whiplash
  B. Fracture of vertebra without dislocation
  C. Fracture of vertebra with dislocation
IV. Treatment
  A. Carefully immobilize head and neck.
  B. Establish airway if needed—usually tracheotomy.
  C. Notify neurosurgeons for treatment—usually tongs and traction.

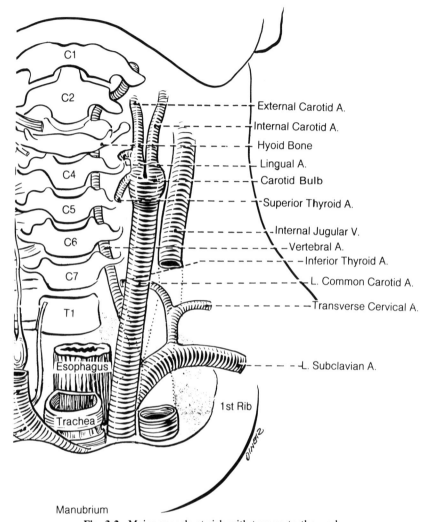

Fig. 3-2. Major vessels at risk with trauma to the neck.

MAJOR VESSELS IN THE NECK

I. Introduction
   A. Major vessels (Figs. 3-2, 3-3)
      1. The major arteries of the neck are the carotid and vertebral arteries with their branches. The innominate artery can ride high into the lower neck and possibly could be injured.
      2. The main veins are the internal jugular veins.

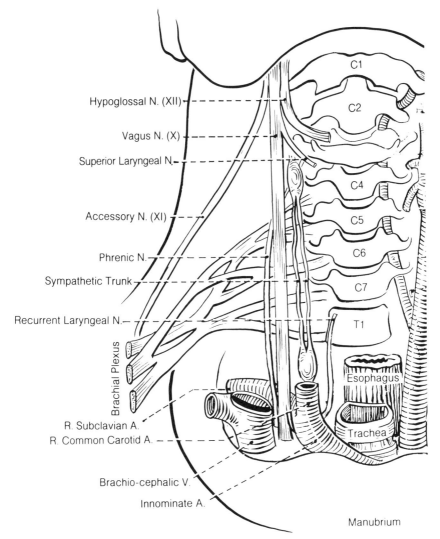

Fig. 3-3. Neurologic structures at risk with neck trauma.

B. Blunt trauma can rupture major vessels, although it is unusual.
C. Penetrating injuries are more likely to injure the vessels.
D. A significant vascular injury may occur without being clinically evident; therefore it is important to have a high degree of suspicion.
E. Assess the trajectory of the missile and try to determine if the trajectory crosses near the path of any of the major vessels.
F. If a major vessel injury is suspected, either explore the wound or, if no emergency exists, do an arteriogram.

II. Differential diagnosis
   A. Soft tissue injury with hematoma
   B. Arterial injury
   C. Jugular vein injury
III. Clinical manifestations
   A. Soft tissue injury with hematoma
       1. Pain
       2. Swelling
       3. Tenderness
       4. Ecchymosis of skin or pharynx
   B. Arterial injury
       1. Marked swelling (usually progressive)
       2. Pain
       3. Tenderness
       4. Ecchymosis of skin or pharynx
       5. Possible airway distress
   C. Jugular vein injury
       1. Swelling (may be progressive)
       2. Pain
       3. Tenderness
       4. Ecchymosis of skin or pharynx
       5. Possible airway distress
IV. Diagnostic studies
   A. Soft tissue x-ray films of neck (AP and lateral) to check trajectory of missile in penetrating neck wounds
   B. Arteriogram
V. Treatment
   A. Soft tissue injury with hematoma: If hematoma is not expanding and there is no airway distress or sign of major blood loss, watchful observation without exploration is the recommended treatment.
   B. Arterial injury[4]: If there is a high degree of suspicion or it is proved by arteriogram, exploration of neck with repair or ligation of vessel is recommended.
   C. Jugular vein injury: If there is a high degree of suspicion or it is proved by arteriogram, exploration of neck with repair or ligation of vessel is recommended.
VI. Complications
   A. Early complications
       1. Shock
       2. Airway obstruction
       3. Stroke
   B. Late complications
       1. Arteriovenous fistula is possible, especially if the carotid and jugular are both injured.
       2. Aneurysm of an artery can occur.

PHARYNX AND ESOPHAGUS

  I. Introduction

The pharynx and esophagus may be lacerated by blunt or penetrating injuries. The injury may not be obvious initially, and because the complications can be fatal it is important to recognize and treat properly.

 II. Differential diagnosis

A. Contusion of the pharynx or esophagus

B. Rupture or laceration of the pharynx or esophagus

III. Clinical manifestations

A. Contusions

1. Usually from blunt trauma

2. Pain

3. Slight or moderate dysphagia

4. Hemoptysis or hematomas

5. Possibly edema or hematomas of the pharynx

6. Mucosal tear without full-thickness laceration, possibly, when the larynx is pushed forcefully against the posterior pharynx

B. Rupture or laceration of the pharynx or esophagus

1. Dysphagia

2. Pain

3. Hemoptysis

4. Subcutaneous emphysema

5. Possibly asymptomatic

6. Untreated injury: usually presents later

a) Fever

b) Odynophagia

c) Abscess formation

d) Mediastinitis

e) Possible edema, hematomas, or lacerations with purulent drainage near the injury

IV. Diagnostic studies

A. AP and lateral soft tissue x-ray films of the neck to look for free air and/or retropharyngeal thickening

B. CT scan to more accurately locate area of injury

C. Direct laryngoscopy and esophagoscopy to localize area of injury. These endoscopy procedures must be performed with caution, as the scopes could cause larger lacerations or false passages.

 V. Treatment

A. Early treatment

1. Closure of lacerations if accessible by laryngoscope

2. Antibiotics

3. Nothing by mouth (if feeding tube needed, inserted under direct visualization)

4. Careful observation

  B. If abscess present or suspected
     1. Neck exploration
     2. Closure of pharynx
     3. Débridement and drainage of wound
     4. Intravenous antibiotics
VI. Complications
  A. Neck abscess
  B. Mediastinitis
  C. Death

NEUROLOGIC STRUCTURES OF THE NECK

  I. Introduction
     There are many neurologic structures in the neck which can be injured
     (Fig. 3-3) and must be considered when trauma has been sustained. Injuries
     can occur from blunt or penetrating trauma.
     A. With blunt trauma the primary structures which can be injured are the
        spinal cord, phrenic nerves (from spinal cord injury), and the recurrent
        laryngeal nerves if laryngotracheal disruption occurs.
     B. Any of the neurologic structures can be damaged with penetrating
        injuries. One must be aware of the major neurologic structures.
 II. Differential diagnosis
     A. Vagus nerve or isolated recurrent laryngeal nerve injury
     B. Spinal accessory nerve injury
     C. Hypoglossal nerve injury
     D. Cervical spinal cord injury
     E. Phrenic nerve injury
     F. Sympathetic plexus injury
     G. Brachial plexus injury
     H. Facial nerve injury
III. Clinical manifestations
     A. Vagus nerve injury
        1. The primary symptom is hoarseness from vocal cord paralysis.
        2. If the injury is above the takeoff of the superior laryngeal nerve,
           there may also be mild aspiration symptoms.
        3. The vocal cord paralysis could also be an isolated recurrent laryn-
           geal nerve injury.
     B. Spinal accessory nerve injury
        1. Dropped shoulder
        2. Difficulty abducting the arm above the head
     C. Hypoglossal nerve injury
        1. Ipsilateral tongue paralysis
        2. Slight dysphagia
        3. Difficulty with articulation

D. Cervical spinal cord injury
   1. Possible spinal shock
   2. Paraplegia or quadriplegia
   3. Dyspnea
E. Phrenic nerve injury
   1. Mild to moderate dyspnea
   2. Decreased breath sounds on involved side
F. Sympathetic plexus injury: Horner's syndrome (miosis, ptosis, anhidrosis)
G. Brachial plexus injury: sensory and motor deficits in the ipsilateral upper extremity
H. Facial nerve injury
   1. Partial or complete paralysis of ipsilateral facial muscles
   2. Occasionally, drooling

IV. Diagnostic studies
   A. Physical examination is probably the most important part of the evaluation.
   B. Signs and symptoms
      1. Vocal cord paralysis (indirect mirror examination)
      2. Shoulder dysfunction
      3. Tongue paralysis
      4. Extremity weakness or paralysis
      5. Decreased breath sounds
      6. Horner's syndrome
      7. Isolated upper extremity sensory or motor deficits
      8. Facial paralysis
   C. Radiographs
      1. To check cervical vertebrae for fractures or dislocations
      2. To check the neck for missile fragments to determine trajectory of penetrating injuries
      3. Chest x-ray film to see diaphragm position

V. Treatment
   A. Vagus nerve injury
      1. A *unilateral* injury does not need to be treated, as the primary problem is vocal cord paralysis and hoarseness, and the patient usually compensates after several months.
      2. With *bilateral* vagus nerve injury[5] the vocal cords are paralyzed close to the midline; and although voice is fairly good, airway obstruction is present because the cords do not abduct. This patient may require a tracheotomy if severe obstruction occurs or could undergo one of several procedures to lateralize a vocal cord or open the glottis more.
      3. Reanastomosis of the vagus nerve is probably not beneficial or successful.

   4. Reanastomosis of a unilateral severed recurrent laryngeal nerve is not recommended.
B. Spinal accessory nerve injury
   1. If not repaired with success, the patient would have mild to moderate disability of the shoulder.
   2. This nerve has a high degree of recovery if reanastomosed or a nerve graft is used.
   3. If the neck is explored for other reasons, reanastomosis or a nerve graft is recommended.
C. Hypoglossal nerve injury
   1. Unilateral tongue paralysis is not usually a severe disability unless the patient uses his or her voice professionally.
   2. The nerve can be reanastomosed with significant probability of some return.
D. Cervical spinal cord injury
   1. Immobilize head and neck.
   2. Assist respirations if indicated.
   3. Treat shock if present.
   4. Notify neurosurgeons for evaluation and treatment.
E. Phrenic nerve injury
   If unilateral and isolated, no treatment is necessary.
F. Sympathetic plexus injury
   1. This usually does not cause major problems and requires no specific treatment.
   2. Miosis is noted if present and is recognized to be associated with this injury rather than a head injury.
G. Brachial plexus injury
   1. If nerves are crushed, no immediate treatment but, rather, observation for degree of spontaneous recovery is recommended.
   2. If nerves are severed, reanastomosis is recommended.
H. Facial nerve injury
   1. Dysfunction is mostly cosmetic, but if upper division is involved the eye on that side is vulnerable to problems.
   2. In most cases, exploration with repair by reanastomosis or a nerve graft is recommended.
VI. Late complications
   A. Vagus nerve injury
      1. Unilateral
         a) Persistent hoarseness
         b) Occasionally, aspiration
      2. Bilateral
         a) Dyspnea on exertion
         b) Airway obstruction
   B. Spinal accessory nerve injury
      1. Severe limitations of movement of shoulder

    2. Moderate to severe pain in shoulder
  C. Hypoglossal nerve injury
    1. Speech difficulties
    2. Swallowing problems
  D. Cervical spinal cord injury
    1. Permanent paralysis of extremities
    2. Bladder dysfunction
  E. Phrenic nerve injury: dyspnea on exertion
  F. Sympathetic plexus injury: usually no significant late complications
  G. Brachial plexus injury
    1. Paralysis of upper extremity
    2. Sensory deficit of upper extremity
  H. Facial nerve injury
    1. Upper division: corneal abrasion, ulcerations, or opacification with loss of vision
    2. Lower division: drooling of saliva and major disfigurement

SUBMANDIBULAR GLAND

I. Introduction

    Trauma to the submandibular gland is of little significance if the hypoglossal nerve, lingual nerve, and mandibularis branch of the facial nerve are not injured. The duct of the gland is seldom injured from a neck wound. The facial artery traverses the gland and must be considered because significant bleeding and hematoma could occur.

II. Treatment
  A. Contusion: no treatment necessary
  B. Laceration: if penetrating wound with no hematoma or nerve injury, observation only
  C. Major tissue loss: submandibular gland resection with exploration of nerves and repair if necessary

THYROID GLAND

I. Introduction

    Trauma to the thyroid gland is unlikely to result in any significant thyroid dysfunction. The major concern is an associated injury of the recurrent laryngeal nerve(s) and bleeding because of the vascularity.

II. Treatment
  A. Contusion: no treatment necessary
  B. Laceration: if penetrating wound with no major bleeding or recurrent nerve injury, observation only
  C. Major tissue loss

1. Explore and débride wound.
2. Attempt to save some of the thyroid gland and one or more of the parathyroid glands.
3. Check for recurrent laryngeal nerve injury and for tracheal and esophageal injury.

REFERENCES

1. Olson NR: Surgical treatment of acute blunt laryngeal injuries. Ann Otol Rhinol Laryngol 87:716, 1978
2. Brantigan CO, Grow JB: Cricothyroidotomy: elective use in respiratory problems requiring tracheostomy. J Thorac Cardiovasc Surg 71:72, 1976
3. Romito MC, Calvin SB, Boyd AD: Cricothyroidotomy—its healing and complications. Surg Forum 28:174, 1977
4. Flint LM, Snyder WH, Perry MO, Shires GT: Management of major vascular injuries in the base of the neck. Arch Surg 106:407, 1973
5. Levine HL, Tucker HM: Surgical management of the paralyzed larynx. In Bailey BJ, Biller HF (eds): Surgery of the Larynx. WB Saunders, St. Louis, 1985

4

Gunshot Wounds to the Face and Neck

James Y. Suen _____

SEVERITY OF INJURY

Gunshot wounds that are immediately fatal usually involve injury to the brain, brain stem, or to major vessels of the head or neck. Patients who survive the immediate trauma usually present in a conscious state and may have significant bleeding or airway obstruction that must be attended to quickly. The seriousness of the injury is dependent upon several factors:

1. Type of weapon and missile
2. Distance of the weapon from the victim
3. Structures injured

Bullet Considerations[1]

The destructive effects of bullets are related to their velocity and mass. The kinetic energy (KE) at impact will determine the capacity to injure, and KE $= \frac{1}{2}$ mass $\times$ velocity^2; therefore, the terminal velocity is relatively more important than mass.

Velocity

See Table 4-1.
I. Bullet velocity is classified as low, under 1000 ft/sec; medium, between 1000 and 2000 ft/sec; and high, over 3000 ft/sec.
II. The higher the velocity the greater the speed the bullet travels through tissues, creating a vacuum effect along the track of the injury.

Mass

I. Semi-jacketed bullet
   The expanding or semi-jacketed bullet expands to two to three times normal size upon impact and is less likely to exit from the patient. Greater

TABLE 4-1. BULLET SPEED

Weapon	Speed (ft/sec)
.38 caliber	800
.45 caliber	860
.22 caliber	1,100
Shotgun	1,200
.357 Magnum	1,500
30/30 Rifle	2,200
M-16	3,200

energy is released into the surrounding tissue and often a cone shaped cavity is created.

II. Full-jacketed bullet

Full-jacketed bullet is commonly used in military weaponry.

A. Tends to travel a longer distance

B. The impact creates a cylindrical cavity and may exit through a large hole.

C. Usually travels at high velocities and creates a large vacuum with secondary shearing and tearing of affected tissues

Action

Bullets will have various amounts of yawing, tumbling, and spiraling actions which affect the nature of the damage produced.

Muzzle-to-Victim Range

Shotgun injuries are related to the muzzle-to-victim range and at close range will cause massive destruction of tissue.

Tissue Considerations[2]

Velocity of Bullet

I. Low velocity

Low velocity wounds tend to be associated with relatively minimal damage related entirely to laceration and crushing effects.

II. High velocity

In general, a high velocity bullet will produce a small entrance and large exit wound.

Tissue Damage

I. Cavity Formation

As a bullet travels through tissues, a cavity is formed. There is some tissue recoil, especially at the points of entry and exit.

II. Effect of Steam

The dissipation of the kinetic energy of the missile produces steam which is contained, under pressure, in the cavity. The pressure effects within the tissues mean that tissue damage extends well beyond the visible track of the missile.

III. Bacterial Infection

Tissue damage and contamination of the wound will predispose the tissues to bacterial infection, especially by anaerobes such as *Clostridium perfringens*.

IV. Bone fragments

When a bullet strikes bone, the kinetic energy is expended and transferred to fragments which act as secondary missiles of much lower velocity.

General Principles of Management

Condition of Patient

I. Unconscious

If a patient is unconscious, examine the rest of the body for other sites of injury.

II. Symptoms of shock

If the patient has symptoms of shock (hypotension and tachycardia), treat appropriately as soon as possible.

Location of Bullet

I. Deep in soft tissue or bone

If a missile or bullet fragment is not causing or expected to cause any problems, then it does not have to be removed.

II. Near surface or major vessel

If a missile or bullet fragment is near a skin or mucosal surface or is near a major vessel, removal should be considered.

GUNSHOT WOUNDS TO THE FACE

It is not uncommon to see a gunshot wound to the face without an injury to the brain or spinal cord, especially with low velocity bullets. Self-inflicted shotgun injuries are frequently not fatal because the end of the shotgun is usually held under the chin with the head hyperextended and the thumb used to push the trigger. This usually results in a facial injury only. However, there is usually massive tissue loss of the face.

Evaluation

History

    I. Type of weapon (pistol, rifle, shotgun)
   II. Direction of missile and distance from weapon
  III. Symptoms of dyspnea, pain, bleeding
  IV. Past history of significant previous illness
   V. Allergies
  VI. Tetanus immunizations

Physical Examination

    I. Check for hemorrhage in the head and neck.
  II. If patient is unconscious, check skull and rest of body for other gunshot wounds or other injuries.
  III. Check for shock symptoms (hypotension and tachycardia).
  IV. Examine eyes for injuries and for dilated pupils.
   V. Evaluate cranial nerves and sympathetic nerves.
  VI. Look for entrance and exit wounds to assess trajectory.

Laboratory Studies

    I. If shocky or if there is significant blood loss, send blood for type and crossmatch.
  II. Obtain CBC, BUN, FBS, and electrolyte levels.

Radiographic Studies

    I. Sinus series (include skull) to locate missile fragments and to evaluate facial bones (Fig. 4-1)
  II. Tape markers on entrance and, if present, the exit wounds.
  III. Computed Tomography (CT scan) with contrast or an arteriogram if time permits and if tests available. These are performed primarily when a vascular injury is suspected.

Treatment: Primarily Emergency[3]

General

I. Check for airway obstruction and alleviate or correct immediately.
II. If bleeding from a skin or mucosal surface, apply pressure, if possible, to control bleeding.
III. Begin intravenous fluids if significant bleeding is suspected.
IV. Type and crossmatch blood.
V. Complete evaluation as outlined above. Assess facial structures involved and extent of injury of each structure.
VI. Treat tetanus prophylactically.
VII. Antibiotics, such as penicillin or erythromycin if allergic to penicillin

Soft Tissue Injuries

I. General
   A. Conservative débridement of damaged tissues and control of bleeding
   B. Closure of skin or mucosal surfaces
      1. Primarily done when there is no involvement of deep tissues that could necrose and cause an abscess.
      2. Should approximate tissues only and tight closures should be avoided.
      3. Drains (Penrose type) may be indicated.
II. Parotid gland
   A. Assess for injury to the facial nerve.
      1. If facial paralysis is present, explore the facial nerve immediately if there are other indications for surgery (such as vascular injury). Should the nerve be partially avulsed, then débride back to healthy nerve and consider a nerve graft.
      2. If facial paralysis is present and there are no other indications for immediate surgical intervention, then surgical exploration could be delayed for several days to allow the injured tissue and nerve to declare themselves. However, after 48 to 72 hours the distal ends of the nerve will no longer be stimulable and therefore the distal ends may be more difficult to identify.
   B. Assess for injury to the parotid (Stenson's) duct.
      1. If injury is suspected, then a lacrimal probe can be used to pass through the parotid duct while the facial wound is inspected for a tear or avulsion.
      2. If significant duct injury is present and primary closure can be accomplished, a small polyethylene tube should be placed in the duct as a stent and sutured in place, then the duct repaired.

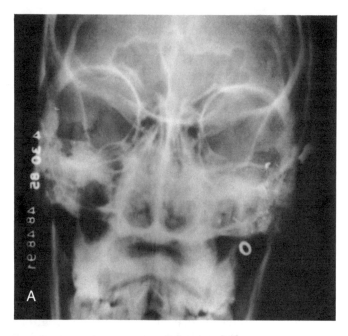

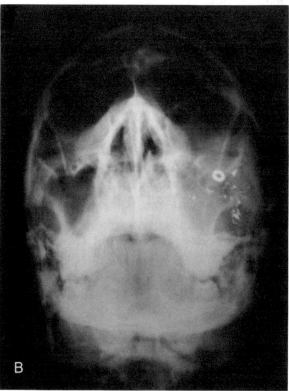

Fig. 4-1. Sinus series with a marker (''0'') taped at the entrance wound to help determine the trajectory and structures injured. (**A**) Caldwell view, (**B**) Waters view.

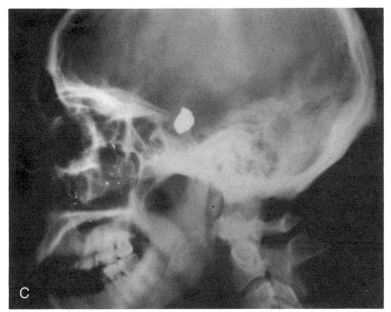

Fig. 4-1. (*continued*) (**C**) Lateral view.

    3. If the duct is not salvageable, then it should be ligated. The parotid gland will swell and may atrophy later or may need to be removed later.

IV. Eye

    Gunshot wounds involving the eye or eyelids should be evaluated by an ophthalmologist.

V. Nose

    Débride wound conservatively. Primary closure should be attempted. Major reconstruction is usually delayed.

VI. Lips

    Débride wound conservatively. Primary closure should be attempted. Major reconstruction is usually delayed.

VII. Tongue

    Débride wound conservatively. Reapproximate tissues loosely.

Bony Injuries[4]

I. Gunshot wounds to the facial bones usually fragment the bones and the pieces can act as secondary missiles so that there may be considerable scatter (Fig. 4-2).

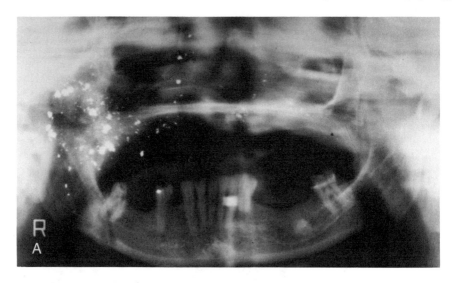

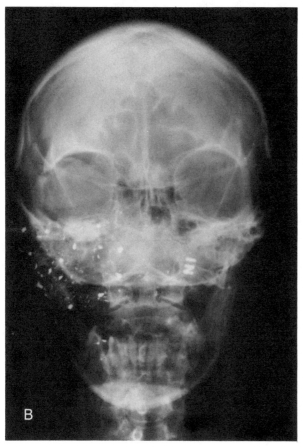

Fig. 4-2. (A) Gunshot wound to the mandible with comminution. The bony fragments can act as secondary missiles. **(B)** Same patient as Fig. 2A with a marker at the entrance wound to help determine trajectory.

II. Orbit

The primary problem with orbital wall involvement is eye injury. Orbital injuries should be seen by an ophthalmologist to decide if surgical exploration is indicated.

III. Midfacial bones

A. With low velocity missile injuries, minimal immediate treatment, e.g., débridement and hemostasis, is indicated.

B. If high velocity missile injury with major tissue and bone loss, treatment would consist of débridement, hemostasis, and approximation of remaining tissues.

C. Facial nerve and parotid duct injuries should be considered and treated appropriately.

D. If large facial skin defect, consider regional flap coverage during the immediate treatment.

E. If the maxillary teeth or the palate is fractured, reduction and intermaxillary fixation should be performed.

F. Maxillary sinus and ethmoid sinus injuries usually do not require much immediate treatment. Delayed treatment such as an ethmoidectomy, nasoantral windows, or Caldwell-Luc procedure of the maxillary sinus may be indicated.

IV. Mandible[5,6]

A. If there is an open wound into the mouth associated with the mandible injury, the mucosal wound should be débrided along with the bony fragments and an attempt made to close the mucosal tears.

B. If teeth are fractured or loose, they may be salvaged by wiring them to adjacent teeth or using an arch bar.

C. Mandible injuries without intraoral communication will usually require débridement externally and, if fractures are present, open reduction and intermaxillary fixation. Frequently the fractured mandible is so comminuted that a biphase (external) appliance is necessary.

D. Bone graft may be indicated later for large bony defects.

Vascular Injuries[7]

I. The internal maxillary artery can be avulsed with significant bleeding into the retropterygoid fossa.

A. With no mucosal tears into the nasopharynx or sinuses, the bleeding usually tamponades itself.

B. With mucosal tears, the bleeding may continue and require packing of the nasopharynx, nose, or sinuses.

C. Occasionally ligation of the internal maxillary artery via a transantral approach or even ligation of the external carotid artery is necessary to control the bleeding.

II. The primary vessels of concern with gunshot wounds to the face are

A. Internal and external carotid arteries

B. The internal jugular vein

III. Patients with suspected injuries to the external or internal carotid arteries or to the internal jugular vein should have arteriograms or CT scans if time permits.
   A. If injury to these vessels is suspected or proven, surgical exploration should be carried out and repair or ligation of the vessels performed.
   B. Any adjacent missile fragments should be removed to prevent erosion into the vessel later.

Shotgun Wounds[8,9]

I. Shotgun wounds to the face cause extensive tissue loss.
II. Self-inflicted shotgun wounds[10] are usually not fatal if the patient does not die of hemorrhage before help arrives. These shotgun blasts usually blow away the mid-chin, mandible, lips, nose, and/or sometimes one or both eyes.
   A. Immediate treatment
      1. Control airway (frequently with tracheotomy).
      2. Control bleeding with pressure and/or ligation.
      3. Débride dead or non-viable soft tissue and loose bone fragments.
      4. Close as much of the remaining tissues as possible, paying attention to the normal anatomical relationships.
      5. Consider external splints to immobilize the remaining mandibular and maxillary bones to maintain normal anatomical relationships.
   B. Delayed treatment is usually extensive and consists of multiple operations for reconstruction, depending upon the defects. This will not be discussed.
III. Shotgun wounds that are not self-inflicted are more often fatal because of central nervous system injuries. If the patient survives, the treatment would be similar to the self-inflicted injury. Large tissue defects on the lateral face may be easier to reconstruct and immediate reconstruction with flaps may be indicated.

GUNSHOT WOUNDS TO THE NECK[11]

Gunshot wounds to the neck are often more dire emergencies than are facial injuries because the airway and major vessels are at greater risk of injury and can be more life-threatening.

Evaluation

History

I. Type of weapon (pistol, rifle, shotgun)
II. Direction of missile and distance from weapon
III. Symptoms of airway obstruction, pain, bleeding

IV. Past history of significant previous illness
 V. Allergies
VI. Tetanus immunizations

Physical Examination

  I. Check for airway obstruction.
 II. Check for active hemorrhage or hematomas of the neck, pharynx, larynx, or trachea.
III. If patient is unconscious, check rest of body for other injuries.
IV. Check for shock symptoms (hypotension and tachycardia).
 V. Look for entrance and exit wounds to assess trajectory.
VI. Evaluate cranial nerves X, XI, and XII, and for Horner's syndrome.
VII. Check for hemiparalysis.
VIII. Check for subcutaneous emphysema.

Laboratory Studies

 I. If patient has symptoms of shock or if there is significant blood loss, send blood for type and crossmatch.
II. Obtain CBC, BUN, FBS, and electrolyte levels.

Radiographic Studies

  I. Anteroposterior and lateral views of the neck and head
 II. Tape markers on entrance and, if present, the exit wounds.
III. Arteriogram or CT scan with contrast if time permits and if available. These are performed primarily when a vascular injury is suspected and the patient is stable.

Treatment

General

 I. Assess airway and if obstruction present, correct immediately (tracheotomy frequently necessary).
II. If bleeding from a surface wound, use pressure to control bleeding.
III. Begin intravenous fluids if significant bleeding suspected; type and crossmatch blood.
IV. Treat tetanus prophylactically.
 V. Antibiotics such as penicillin, or erythromycin if allergic to penicillin.

Larynx or Trachea Injury

I. Look for airway distress and subcutaneous emphysema.
II. Tracheotomy
III. Will usually require surgical exploration with repair of injuries and possibly a stent to prevent stenosis and maintain airway

Vascular Injuries[12-14]

I. The primary vessels of concern are the common carotid, internal and external carotid, and vertebral arteries and the internal jugular vein (Fig. 4-3).

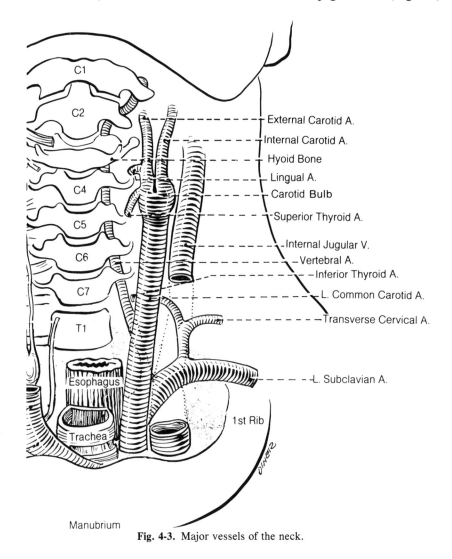

Fig. 4-3. Major vessels of the neck.

II. In the lower neck on the right the innominate artery may be located high enough to be injured. Also the thyrocervical trunk and its branches can be injured.

III. The branches of the external carotid can cause troublesome bleeding.

IV. If a hematoma is progressive and causing airway problems, then immediate exploration is indicated. Most vessels can be ligated. If upon ligation of the vertebral, common carotid, or internal carotid artery the patient has obvious neurological problems, then arterial repair with or without a graft should be considered.

Pharynx or Esophagus Injury[15]

When obvious injuries to these structures are present, surgical exploration via the neck is usually indicated with attempted repair of the mucosal wall and adequate wound drainage through the skin incision.

Neurological Injuries

I. With spinal cord injury the patient's neck should be immobilized and a neurosurgeon notified to see the patient.

II. If injury of the spinal accessory nerve or brachial plexus nerves is present, an attempt to reanastomose the nerve(s) may be indicated.

III. Unilateral injury of the hypoglossal, vagus, phrenic, sympathetics, or recurrent laryngeal nerves is usually not significant and no repair is indicated.

Cervical Spine Injuries[16]

I. Fracture and/or dislocation should be identified. The neck should be immobilized and a neurosurgeon notified.

II. When gunshot wounds to the cervical spine occur and are associated with a pharyngeal wound, the bullet should be considered for removal because the incidence of osteomyelitis is high and the complications major.

III. When bullets lodge in the cervical spine with no associated mucosal injury and no significant symptoms or problems, the bullet does not necessarily have to be removed.

REFERENCES

1. Emergency War Surgery, 1st Revision. p. 9. Fundamentals of wound ballistics. Department of Defense, Government Printing Office, Washington, DC, 1975
2. DeMuth WE, Smith JM: High-velocity bullet wounds of muscle and bone: the basis of rational early treatment. J Trauma 6:744, 1966

3. Broadbent TR, Woolf RM: Gunshot wounds of the face: initial care. J Trauma 12:229, 1972
4. Rowe NL, Williams JL: Maxillofacial Injuries, Vol. 2. Churchill Livingstone, London, 1985
5. May M, Cutchavaree A, Chadaratana P: Mandibular fractures from civilian gunshot wounds: A study of 20 cases. Laryngoscope 83:969, 1973
6. Lucas JW, Georgen GJ, Monaco F: Management of shotgun wounds of the symphysis. J Oral Surg 33:623, 1975
7. Banks P, Redpath TH: Closed carotid artery hemorrhage as a complication of minor gunshot wounds of the face and jaws. J Oral Surg 30:176, 1972
8. Sherman RT, Parrish RA: Management of shotgun injuries: A review of 152 cases. J Trauma 3:76, 1963
9. Spira M, Hardy SB, Biggs TE, Gerow FJ: Shotgun injuries of the face. Plas Reconstr Surg 39:449, 1967
10. Nordenram A, Freiberg N: Suicidal gunshot wounds resulting in severe maxillofacial injury. Intl J Oral Surg 3:29, 1974
11. May M, Tucker HM, Dillard BM: Penetrating wounds of the neck in civilians. Otolaryngol Clin N Amer 9:361, 1976
12. Flint LM, Snyder WH, Perry MO, Shires GT: Management of major vascular injuries in the base of the neck. Arch Surg 106:407, 1973
13. May M, Lee C, Sapote C, et al: Penetrating wounds of the neck: selective exploration. A study of 100 cases. Trans Am Acad Ophthalmol Otolaryngol 75:497, 1971
14. Shirkey AL, Beall AC, DeBakey ME: Surgical management of penetrating wounds of the neck. Arch Surg 86:955, 1963
15. Popousky J, Lee YC, Berk JL: Gunshot wounds of the esophagus. J Thor Cardiovasc Surg 72:609, 1976
16. Schaefer SD, Bucholz RW, Jones RE, Carder HM. The management of transpharyngeal gunshot wounds to the cervical spine. Surg Gynecol Obst 152:27, 1981

5

Ear Infections

Robert W. Seibert _____

Infections of the external and middle ear constitute one of the most frequent problems in medical practice. It has been determined that otitis media is the most common illness for which a child consults a physician.[1] Often such infections produce severe pain or high fevers that necessitate emergent treatment. Because of the intimate anatomic and physiologic relations of the middle ear to the inner ear and intracranial structures, an improper or delayed diagnosis may lead to serious sequelae, even death.

In addition to acute infections, middle ear disease may remain quiescent for many years and manifest its presence only with the onset of a severe, possibly life-threatening complication. It is beyond the scope of this chapter to comprehensively discuss the problem of otitis media; however, physicians must be familiar with the diagnosis and management of the emergency aspects of these important infections.

EXTERNAL EAR

I. The external ear consists of the auricle or pinna and external auditory canal. The structure of the auricle is a delicate scrollwork of elastic cartilage covered by a thin layer of subcutaneous fat and skin.

II. Because the auricle is in a relatively exposed position on the head it is frequently subjected to trauma. Infection of traumatized tissue may result in perichondritis or chondritis.

III. The external auditory canal consists of an outer cartilaginous portion and an inner bony portion lined by thin skin without appendages. This medial skin is tightly adherent to the underlying bone so that trauma or infection produces severe pain.

Perichondritis and Chondritis of the Auricle

I. Infection of the auricular soft tissues (perichondritis) or cartilage (chondritis) may follow trauma, including surgery, and severe external otitis.

II. Signs and symptoms
   A. Painful and swollen auricle

65

B. May drain serous to seropurulent material from areas of skin breakdown

C. Early edema and inflammation of auricular skin

D. With chronic infection, the skin becomes thickened and erythematous, with possible areas of necrosis and purulent drainage.

E. Signs of a severe infection may indicate extension of infection to the cartilage with destruction of auricular cartilage.

III. Treatment

A. Prophylaxis

1. Treat external otitis and surrounding cellulitis with oral or parenteral antibiotics.

2. Auricular hematomas are aspirated or incised and drained; antibiotic coverage is begun.

3. Lacerations involving the cartilage receive prophylactic antibiotic coverage.

B. Treatment of perichondritis consists of high-dose intravenous antibiotics covering the usual pathogenic gram-positive bacteria as well as gram-negative organisms (see treatment of severe external otitis, below). In the absence of cartilage involvement, improvement should be noted in 24 to 48 hours.

C. Because cartilage has poor blood supply, once infection is established control by medical means alone is usually ineffective. Surgical débridement is required to remove irreversibly infected cartilage. The diagnosis of chondritis frequently depends on failure of clinical response to antibiotic treatment.

D. Failure of improvement with medical treatment usually requires incision and drainage of any abscess, as well as débridement of necrotic cartilage back to healthy tissue. The final result is frequently a severely deformed auricle.

Furuncle in the External Auditory Canal

I. Etiology

Furuncles occur in the cartilaginous canal where the skin contains appendages. *Staphylococcus aureus* is the most likely organism.

II. Signs and symptoms

A. Pain and tenderness are experienced on motion of the auricle.

B. The localized, inflamed furuncle is usually obvious on inspection.

C. No drainage is present unless the lesion has ruptured.

III. Treatment

A. Local heat and topical antibiotic ointment or drops are usually effective.

B. Systemic antibiotics with antistaphylococci coverage are helpful in severe cases (dicloxacillin 25 mg/kg in four doses in children and 250 mg every 6 hours in adults or cephalexin 100 mg/kg in four doses in children and 250 to 500 mg every 6 hours in adults).

C. Incision and drainage may be necessary if frank abscess develops.

D. Analgesics are indicated for pain relief.

External Otitis

I. Etiology

Infection of the external auditory canal is predisposed by several factors.

A. Environment: The external auditory canal is warm and moist.

B. Normal bacterial flora within the external auditory canal usually includes potential pathogens, especially *Pseudomonas aeruginosa* and *Staphylococcus*.

C. Damage to the external auditory canal skin, as with traumatic removal of excess cerumen, can cause infection.

D. Water exposure, e.g., swimming, can result in maceration of the skin, bacterial proliferation, invasion, and clinical infection.

II. Signs and symptoms

A. Pain is frequently severe, especially on palpation or motion of the auricle.

B. There is marked tenderness when pressure is applied to the tragus of the ear, as well as pain on motion of the auricle.

C. External canal skin is inflamed and edematous.

D. Otorrhea varies from serous to purulent or may be absent. *Pseudomonas* infection may produce a greenish-blue discharge with a sickly sweet odor reminiscent of grapes. Foul-smelling fecal odor is produced by infections with *Proteus* or anaerobes.

E. Hearing loss may be nonexistent to mild and is due to obstruction from cerumen, otorrhea, or edema.

F. In severe infections cellulitis may extend beyond the external auditory canal to the auricle and surrounding tissues.

G. Periauricular lymph nodes, especially preauricular, may be enlarged and tender.

III. Treatment

Treatment of external otitis is divided into local and systemic approaches. More severe infections require a combination of the two.

A. Local infection

1. External auditory canal cleansing. Careful cleaning of the external auditory canal with removal of exudate allows the topical agents to reach infected skin. Gentle irrigations may be helpful.

2. Topical solutions containing antibiotics singly or in combination with a steroid compound. The antibiotic agents usually used are Chloromycetin, gentamicin, or a combination of polymixin and neomycin. Cortisporin Otic Suspension is effective and commonly used. Otic solutions containing acetic acid (Vosol) may also be effective. Topical agents used in the form of otic drops are applied three or four times per day for 7 to 10 days.

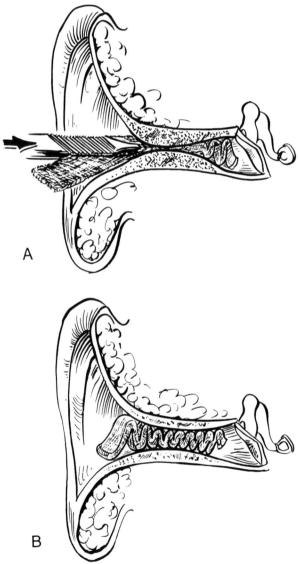

Fig. 5-1. (A) A gauze wick moistioned with ear drops is gently inserted into the ear canal. (B) The wick mechanically compresses the edema and serves as a conduit for ear drops.

   3. External auditory canal wick (Fig. 5-1). Frequently the external auditory canal is swollen so that otic drops cannot penetrate the canal. If this occurs, after gentle removal of exudate in the canal, a cotton or synthetic commercially available wick may be placed to serve as a route for topical agents. Ideally, the wick extends close to the tympanic membrane. The wick may also compress edema from the external auditory canal skin. Insertion of a wick is quite uncomfortable for the patient and requires great care and gentleness. The wick is changed every 1 to 2 days until the external auditory canal lumen is large enough to allow penetration of drops. Usually the wick extrudes when the edema subsides.
   4. Water precautions. The patient should avoid water contacting the external auditory canal during acute infections.
B. Systemic infection
   Systemic antibiotics are indicated in severe infections when there is extension beyond the external auditory canal. Culture of exudate is mandatory. Initial treatment includes both anti-*Pseudomonas* (gentamicin 3 to 5 mg/kg in adults, and 5 to 7 mg/kg in children over 24 hours in three doses) and anti-*Staphylococcus* coverage (nafcillin 50 to 100 mg/kg 24 hours in four to six doses).

"Malignant" External Otitis

 I. Pathophysiology
    A. A chronic osteitis of the temporal bone in patients with diabetes mellitus
    B. Usually caused by *Pseudomonas aeruginosa*
II. Signs and symptoms
    A. Otalgia, especially of a deep nature
    B. Otorrhea
    C. Classically, erosion of the floor of the external auditory canal with granulation tissue at the bone–cartilage junction
    D. Facial nerve paralysis often with progressive infection of the temporal bone
    E. Later, possibly multiple cranial nerve deficits and meningitis resulting in death
III. Treatment
    A. Extensive surgical débridement of the infected site in the external auditory canal or partial temporal bone resection is recommended.
    B. Six weeks of high-dose intravenous antibiotics, usually carbenicillin (400 to 500 mg/kg/24 hours) and gentamicin (3 to 5 mg/kg in adults and 5 to 7 mg/kg in children, over 24 hours), is indicated.
    C. Inadequate treatment results in high mortality.

MIDDLE EAR AND MASTOID

Middle ear infections are extremely prevalent, particularly in the pediatric age group. For comprehensive treatment of the subject the reader is referred to Bluestone and Stool.[2]

The nomenclature of middle ear disease is varied and confusing, e.g., "serous otitis media," "secretory otitis media," "glue ear," "suppurative otitis media." An acceptable generic term is "otitis media with effusion," with the adjectives "acute" or "chronic" being applied when indicated.

Two principal factors in the development of middle ear and mastoid disease appear to be eustachian tube dysfunction and middle ear infection. The local immune mechanism of the middle ear and allergy undoubtedly play roles in many patients.[3]

Acute Otitis Media

I. Etiology
   A. Predisposing factors
      1. Most common between 6 and 24 months of age
      2. More common in male patients than female patients
      3. Increased incidence in American Indians and Eskimos
      4. Most common during winter and spring
      5. Preceding viral upper respiratory tract infections
      6. Altered host defenses as seen in cleft palate
      7. Immunologic deficiences
      8. Malignancy
   B. Microbiology
      1. Bacteria: most common pathogenic organisms are *Streptococcus pneumoniae* and *Hemophilus influenzae*. Group A *Streptococcus* and *Staphylococcus aureus* may be responsible but are not as common.[4]
      2. Viruses are rarely found (respiratory syncytial and influenza viruses most common)[5] but may be the initial insult in an episode of bacterial otitis media.
      3. *Mycoplasma* has been found to cause bullous myringitis with hemorrhage and bleb formation in the tympanic membrane. Most cases are due to viruses, as several studies fail to show an increase in *Mycoplasma* titers in bullous myringitis.[6]
      4. *Chlamydia*: otitis media due to *Chlamydia trachomatis* may occur in infants less than 6 months of age, especially when lower respiratory infection is present.
II. Signs and symptoms

A. Otalgia: Pain is frequently but not invariably present. Severe pain is most common with pneumococcus infection[7] but is also experienced in bullous myringitis.

B. Otorrhea: Seropurulent to purulent discharge with bloody component is commonly seen at the time of spontaneous tympanic membrane perforation.

C. Hearing loss is usually in the mild, occasionally moderate, range.

D. Pulling or rubbing on the ear is common in infants and young children.

E. Irritability may be the only symptom in infants.

F. Fever is variable. High fever with febrile seizures is associated with *Streptococcus pneumoniae* infections.[7]

G. Anorexia, vomiting, and/or diarrhea may occur in infants and young children with acute otitis media.

H. Auricular and tragal tenderness is not present unless there is associated external otitis.

I. Otoscopy
   1. Tympanic membrane intact
      a) Tympanic membrane injected; may be only sign in mild infection
      b) Inflamed tympanic membrane; may show hemorrhagic areas
      c) Bulging tympanic membrane: localized or diffuse
      d) Loss of landmarks
      e) Vesicles or blebs on tympanic membrane in bullous myringitis
      f) Air–fluid level or bubbles behind tympanic membrane; more common in chronic effusion
      g) Sluggish mobility of tympanic membrane
   2. Tympanic membrane perforated
      a) Perforation
      b) Otorrhea

III. Tests

A. Tympanography shows a flat or barely rounded curve (type B tympanogram).

B. Tuning fork
   1. Weber test: Hold vibrating tuning fork on midline of forehead. Sound lateralizes to the ear with the conductive hearing loss.
   2. Rinne test: Compare loudness of tuning fork when it is held beside ear (air conduction) to when it is placed on mastoid bone behind ear (bone conduction). The tuning fork is heard more loudly by bone conduction than by air conduction in the presence of a conductive hearing loss as seen with otitis media.

C. Audiogram shows a conductive hearing loss usually in the mild to moderate range.

D. X-ray examination: Mastoid x-ray films are rarely indicated unless a complication such as coalescent mastoiditis is suspected. In acute suppurative otitis media the mastoid air cell system may be filled with exudate and inflamed mucosa, and it appears opacified on x-ray films.

Bony septae between air cells appear intact. Loss of septae is suggestive of a coalescent or surgical mastoiditis. This complication is an indication for surgery (mastoidectomy).

IV. Differential diagnosis
  A. Injected tympanic membrane in febrile or crying child
  B. External otitis. If the tympanic membrane cannot be adequately visualized in external otitis and suppurative otitis media cannot be definitely ruled out, the more significant infection, i.e., otitis media, is treated.
  C. Nonsuppurative otitis media
    1. Signs and symptoms
      a) Tympanic membrane is dull, frequently retracted, and poorly mobile.
      b) Injection is minimal, but often the tympanic membrane is orange.
      c) An air–fluid level or bubble may be present.
    2. Treatment
      a) Antibiotics: see treatment of acute otitis media.
      b) Decongestants and antihistamines
      c) Eustachian tube exercises
      d) Myringotomy and ventilating tube insertion
      e) Possibly adenoidectomy[2]
V. Treatment of acute otitis media
  A. Medical treatment
     Although most cases of acute otitis media resolve spontaneously, antimicrobial agents speed resolution and almost eliminate the incidence of suppurative complications.[2]
    1. Oral antibiotics—pediatric doses
      a) Ampicillin 50 to 100 mg/kg/24 hours in four divided doses for 10 days, *or*
      b) Amoxicillin 40 mg/kg/24 hours in three divided doses for 10 days
      c) Both of these agents are active against *S. pneumoniae* and *H. influenza* (non-β-lactamase-producing strains).
      d) If patient is allergic to penicillin
        (1) Erythromycin 40 mg/kg/24 hours and sulfisoxazole 120 mg/kg/24 hours in four divided doses, *or*
        (2) The fixed combination (Pediazole)
      e) If a resistant strain of *H. influenzae* is suspected because of failure of initial therapy or is found on tympanocentesis culture results
        (1) Erythromycin–sulfisoxazole combination as above, *or*
        (2) Trimethoprim 8 mg/kg/24 hours and sulfamethoxazole 40 mg/kg/24 hours (Bactrim or Septra) in two divided doses, *or*
        (3) Cefaclor 40 mg/kg/24 hours in three divided doses, *or*

(4) Augmentin, a drug combining amoxicillin and clavulanic acid, a β-lactamase inhibitor, 20 to 40 mg/kg/24 hours in three divided doses

2. Parenteral antibiotics: For the patient who is vomiting or unable to take oral medication, use intramuscular benzathine penicillin.

a) Patient less than 30 pounds: 600,000 units in one dose; more than 30 pounds, 1,200,000 units in one dose; combine with sulfisoxazole to cover *H. influenzae*.

b) Neonate: Different dosage schedules apply because of different physiologic processes of the newborn. The reader is advised to consult specific references.[8]

3. Topical antibiotic–steroid otic solutions may be used in the ear when there is tympanic membrane perforation and otorrhea; they may also be used in bullous myringitis.

4. Antihistamine–decongestants. Systemic agents may produce symptomatic relief; however, there is little if any evidence that these drugs, especially topical decongestants, influence the course of the disease.[9]

B. Surgical treatment

1. Myringotomy

a) Severe otalgia unresponsive to narcotic analgesics

b) Fever unresponsive to antibiotics, acetaminophen, or aspirin

c) Although there is little evidence that a myringotomy hastens resolution of the acute inflammatory process,[10] it may decrease the likelihood of persistent middle ear effusion.[8]

2. Myringotomy and tympanocentesis with culture of the middle ear

a) Otitis media in seriously ill or toxic patient

b) Otitis media in newborn or immunologically compromised patient

c) Otitis media in patient already receiving antibiotic or clinical response failure to antibiotics.[2]

3. Myringtomy and insertion of ventilation tube

a) Presence of facial nerve paralysis secondary to inflammation of the facial nerve in its course through the middle ear

b) Acute vertigo due to serous labyrinthitis. In these cases surgical treatment consists in drainage of the middle ear space either by wide myringotomy alone or, preferably, myringotomy and insertion of a ventilating tube.

Coalescent Mastoiditis

I. General considerations

A. Seen as an extension of otitis media into the mastoid air cell system with an abscess and destruction of bone

    B. Usually follows a bout of acute otitis media of 2 weeks' or longer duration

II. Signs and symptoms

    A. Recurrence of ear pain after several days of improvement during a bout of acute otitis media

    B. Inflamed, thickened tympanic membrane, often with a perforation that is draining purulent material

    C. Edematous sagging of the posterior-superior external auditory canal skin due to the proximity of this area to the mastoid antrum

    D. Fluctuant abscess with protruding auricle if there is extension through the lateral mastoid cortex

    E. Mastoid x-rays films reveal loss of bony septae with a "ground glass" appearance of the mastoid.

III. Treatment

    A. Intravenous antibiotics—pediatric doses

        1. Recent infection: ampicillin 200 to 300 mg/kg/24 hours in four to six doses (other than neonates)

        2. Persistent infection or resistant infection

            a) Gentamicin 5 to 7.5 mg/kg/24 hours in three doses, *and*

            b) Oxacillin, nafcillin, or methicillin 200 mg/kg/24 hours in four to six doses

    B. Mastoidectomy

        Complete mastoidectomy is done to provide wide drainage and removal of irreversibly infected soft tissue and bone.

IV. Complications

    A. Bezold's abscess, a mass along the sternocleidomastoid muscle in the neck

    B. Intracranial complications

        1. Subdural, epidural, or brain abscess

        2. Meningitis

        3. Focal encephalitis

        4. Lateral sinus thrombophlebitis

        5. Otitic hydrocephalus

REFERENCES

1. Ambulatory Medical Care Rendered in Pediatricians' Offices During 1975 (Advance Date No. 13). National Center for Health Statistics, Hyattsville, MD, 1977
2. Bluestone CD, Stool SE (eds): Pediatric Otolaryngology. Vol. I. p. 85. WB Saunders, Philadelphia, 1983
3. Senturia BH, Bluestone CD, Lim DJ, Saunders WH (eds): Recent advances in otitis media with effusion. Ann Otol Rhinol Laryngol, 89:suppl. 68, 1980
4. Shurin PA, Howie VM, Pelton SI, et al: Bacterial etiology of otitis media during the first six weeks of life. J Pediatr 92:89, 1978

5. Klein JO, Teele DW: Isolation of viruses and mycoplasmas from middle ear effusions: a review. Ann Otol Rhinol Laryngol 85:140, 1976

6. Sobeslavsky O, Syrucck L, Bruckoya M, Abrahanovic M: The etiological role of Mycoplasma pneumoniae in otitis media in children. Pediatrics 35:652, 1965

7. Howie VM, Ploussard JH, Lester RC: Otitis media: a clinical and bacteriological correlation. Pediatrics 45:29, 1970

8. Quarnberg Y, Palva T: Active and conservative treatment of acute otitis media: prospective studies. Ann Otol Rhinol Laryngol, 89:suppl. 68:312, 1980

9. Cantekin EZ, Bluestone CD, Rockette HE, Beery QC: Effect of decongestant with or without antihistamine on eustachian tube function. Ann Otol Rhinol Laryngol, 89:suppl. 68:290, 1980

10. Roddey OF Jr, Earle N Jr, Haggerty R: Myringotomy in acute otitis media: a controlled study. JAMA 197:849, 1966

6

Upper Aerodigestive Tract Infections

Nancy L. Snyderman ⎯⎯⎯⎯⎯⎯⎯⎯⎯⎯⎯⎯⎯⎯⎯

Infections of the upper aerodigestive tract account for more patient visits to the family practitioner, emergency room physician, and otolaryngologist than any other group of ailments. Consequently, it is important for the primary physician to be able to diagnose and treat these problems correctly and expediently. Fortunately, the majority are not life-threatening, although they may cause significant morbidity from temporary impairment and from the disruption of everyday activities.

RHINITIS

Allergic Rhinitis

In allergic rhinitis the nose serves as the end organ for the reaction of antigens with previously formed antibodies. This reaction is mediated by immunoglobulin E (IgE). Allergic rhinitis may vary from season to season and in the most complicated cases may be perennial.

I. Signs and symptoms
   A. Sneezing
   B. Nasal obstruction
   C. Conjunctivitis
   D. Itching of the medial aspect of the eye
   E. Watery rhinorrhea
   F. Congested, blue-gray or purple, wet turbinates and nasal mucosa
   G. Enlargement of inferior turbinate
   H. Pharyngeal irritation
   I. "Allergic salute"—constant, upward rubbing of the nose causing a transverse crease just above the nasal tip

II. Diagnosis
   A. History
   B. Skin testing
   C. Serologic tests (RAST, PRIST, immunoperoxidase)

III. Treatment

A. Acute treatment: directed toward relieving the symptoms. This can best be achieved with antihistamines, decongestants, and sometimes a short course of steroids. Hydrocortisone in a dosage of 50 to 100 mg each day may be effective. Topical nasal steroid sprays (beclomethasone) may also be of benefit.
B. Long-term treatment: directed at eliminating the offending allergin
   1. Early spring: tree pollen
   2. Late spring or early summer (May to June): primarily grasses
   3. Fall (mid-August until frost): ragweed pollen
C. If a patient can isolate symptoms to a particular season, he is directed to an allergist for a thorough evaluation. Some patients exhibit symptoms during all seasons and may need allergy testing for foods as well as for inhalants. Only after this approach can appropriate immunotherapy be started.

Vasomotor Rhinitis

Vasomotor rhinitis is a complex exaggeration of the normal nasal cycle. Powerful vasodilators are released. The most ubiquitous and important mediator is acetylcholine. Allergies, emotional changes, and alterations in temperature and humidity have been implicated as stimuli.

I. Signs and symptoms
   A. Nasal obstruction
   B. Increased watery nasal secretions
   C. Sneezing, particularly in the morning
   D. Pale, boggy, edematous nasal mucosa
   E. Rarely, seasonal variation
II. Treatment
   A. Antihistamines
   B. Inhalant steroids
   C. Steroid injection of the inferior turbinates
   D. Submucosal diathermy
   E. Vidian neurectomy is controversial

Infectious Rhinitis

For both acute and chronic sinusitis, see below. For foreign body-induced rhinitis, see Chapter 13.

Rhinitis Medicamentosa

Rhinitis medicamentosa results from the abuse of nasal sprays and topical decongestants and is frequently overlooked as a cause of nasal obstruction.

I. Signs and symptoms
   A. Nasal stuffiness
   B. Profuse, watery nasal secretions
   C. Erythematous, inflamed, congested turbinates
II. Diagnosis
   The diagnosis is made by a thorough history with particular attention paid to medication use.
III. Treatment
   A. Discontinuation of nasal sprays and decongestants
   B. Oral steroids in tapering dosage
   C. Inhalant steroids
   D. Normal saline nosedrops

SINUSITIS

Any interference with the natural outflow tract of the sinuses may cause obstruction, inspissation of secretions, stagnation, and secondary infection. This can result from a deviated septum, nasal polyps, foreign body, trauma, or a proceeding upper respiratory infection.

Acute Sinusitis

See Fig. 6-1.

Acute Frontal Sinusitis

There is no correlation between the size of the frontal sinus and recognized or unrecognized infections. The frontal sinuses first appear between the ages of 6 to 8 and become fully developed by age 10.[1] They are the most variable sinuses and do not develop at all in a small portion of the population. *Pneumoccoccus* and *Hemophilus influenzae* are the most common organisms found.[2]

I. Signs and symptoms
   The symptoms vary in proportion to the extent of obstruction of the nasofrontal duct.
   A. Severe frontal headache. This is usually over the frontal sinus but may also present as pain behind the eyes. Pain is constant and is exacerbated by palpation of the frontal sinus.
   B. Pain on palpation or percussion of the frontal sinus. The best place to palpate is inferior and medial on the supraorbital rim over the area of the nasofrontal duct.
   C. Thick mucopurulent secretions in the middle meatus

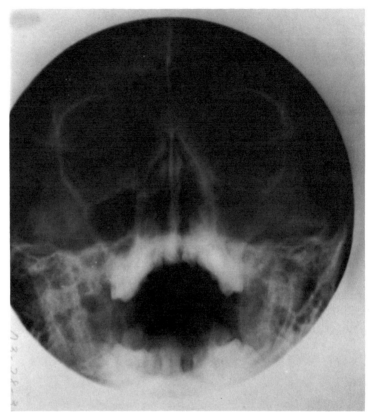

Fig. 6-1. Bilateral frontal sinusitis with an air–fluid level and left maxillary sinusitis.

    D. Low-grade fever

    E. Malaise

    F. Upper eyelid edema in severe cases of acute frontal sinusitis

 II. X-ray examination

    A Caldwell x-ray film is the best view of the frontal sinus. Acute infection may result in complete opacification, an air–fluid level, or mucosal thickening.

III. Treatment

    A. Antibiotics are administered immediately. The drug of choice is amoxicillin.

    B. Spray nasal decongestants are given for 24 to 48 hours to open the nasofrontal duct. By opening this duct, some relief is noted secondary to improved drainage of the frontal sinus.

    C. Oral decongestants for 5 to 7 days

    D. Analgesics

    E. Surgical trephine drainage if the air–fluid level and pain or fever do not improve within 48 hours.
IV. Complications
    A. Frontal osteitis
    B. Mucocele or pyocele
    C. Frontal lobe abscess
    D. Meningitis

Acute Maxillary Sinusitis

Acute maxillary sinusitis is a very common disease. The maxillary sinuses are present at birth and may cause significant problems in the pediatric patient as well as in the adult.
  I. Signs and symptoms
    A. Pain over the cheeks, nose, or teeth; usually dull, aching, or throbbing and may be accentuated by leaning over
    B. Headache
    C. Malaise
    D. Fever
    E. Nasal obstruction
    F. Mucopurulent secretions
    G. Mucosal congestion and erythema
 II. Diagnosis
    X-ray studies are not essential for the diagnosis and treatment of the clear-cut case but may aid in the patient with few clinical clues. A Waters view is the best for demonstrating an air–fluid level. Complete opacification may also be seen in a Caldwell view.
III. Treatment
    A. Antibiotics are administered immediately. The drug of choice is amoxicillin.
    B. Nasal spray decongestants are given for 24 to 48 hours to open the draining meatus. By opening the middle meatus, some relief is noted secondary to improved drainage of the frontal sinus. Oral decongestants may be given simultaneously for 5 to 7 days.
    C. Analgesics are given as needed.
    D. Antral puncture for drainage if the air–fluid level and pain or fever do not improve within 48 hours. Irrigation is not performed in the presence of an acute infection for fear of secondary septic emboli.

Acute Ethmoiditis

Acute ethmoiditis is the most common type of sinus infection in the pediatric age group. The ethmoid sinuses are present at birth. Because of the thin lateral wall, the lamina papyracea of the orbit, ethmoid sinusitis has a predilection for spreading to surrounding soft tissues, especially the orbit.

I. Signs and symptoms
   A. Headache, located between and behind the eyes and sometimes radiating to the temporal area
   B. Tenderness over the medial aspect of the eye
   C. Nasal obstruction
   D. Purulent nasal discharge with posterior nasal drip. Pus may be seen in the middle meatus.
   E. Erythematous, congested nasal mucosa
   F. Fever
   G. Malaise
   H. Periorbital swelling, erythema, and chemosis
II. X-ray examination
    Submentovertex, Caldwell, and Waters views are good for visualizing the ethmoid sinuses. When infected, the sinuses appear cloudy. *Note:* Beware not to diagnose acute ethmoiditis in an infant who has been crying and lying on his back during exposure of the x-ray film. This behavior causes reflux of nasal secretions into the ethmoid air cells and can mimic an acute process.
III. Treatment
    A. Antibiotics: amoxicillin 125 mg p.o. q8h for children less than 10 kg and 250 mg q8h for patients greater than 10 kg
    B. Humidification
    C. Oral decongestants for 5 to 7 days
    D. Nasal spray for 48 hours
IV. Complications—See also Chapter 7, Periorbital Area
    Acute ethmoiditis may lead to orbital and central nervous system (CNS) complications if not treated appropriately and early. Complications in order of increasing severity include:
    A. Periorbital cellulitis
    B. Orbital cellulitis
    C. Retrograde thrombophlebitis
    D. Orbital abscess
    E. Meningitis
    F. Cavernous sinus thrombosis
If any of these occur after appropriate oral antibiotic therapy, then hospitalization, intravenous antibiotics, and possible surgical intervention should follow. An orbital abscess may be drained via an ethmoidectomy approach.

Acute Sphenoiditis

The sphenoid sinus is the least often involved and is a rare site for an isolated infection.
    I. Signs and symptoms

A. Headache. The pain is usually occipital. It is constant and may be severe. Classically, patients describe the pain to be "behind the eye."
B. Purulent postnasal discharge. Secretions appear in the superior meatus and the sphenoethmoid recess.
C. Low-grade fever is present.
D. In severe cases, ophthalmologic changes can result, including proptosis, scotomas, and optic nerve encroachment with fluctuating vision.
II. X-ray examination
The sphenoid sinus, which can be seen on a lateral or submental vertex x-ray film, may exhibit opacification, an air–fluid level, or thickening of the mucous membrane.
III. Treatment
A. Antibiotics: amoxicillin
B. Nasal decongestants
C. Analgesics
D. Surgical drainage if medical therapy is not effective

Chronic Sinusitis

Chronic Frontal Sinusitis

Chronic frontal sinusitis usually results from repeated episodes of acute sinusitis. The end result is thickening of the mucous membranes with obstruction of the nasofrontal duct. There is a tendency of the epithelium to stratify, similar to squamous epithelium, and the mucous membrane loses its proper function.
I. Signs and symptoms
A. Minimal pain and headache. Most patients complain of a fullness in the frontal area.
B. Purulent nasal discharge
II. X-ray examination
Frontal x-ray films may show thickening of the mucous membrane lining the wall of the sinus with sclerosis of the bony margins. Secondary bone destruction may be seen in advanced cases. Late findings may be pyoceles or mucopyoceles.
III. Treatment
Treatment is surgical. The approach is external with a coronal or a brow incision. The aim of the operation is to eradicate all the mucous membrane of the frontal sinus and occlude the nasofrontal ducts in order to prevent further seeding of bacteria from the nose.
IV. Complications
A. Frontal osteitis (Pott's puffy tumor)
B. Mucocele or pyocele
C. Frontal lobe abscess
D. Meningitis

Chronic Maxillary Sinusitis

Chronic maxillary sinusitis results from repeated bouts of an acute process. It may stem from dental origin, and great care is taken to inspect the mouth.
  I. Signs and symptoms
     A. Pressure in the medial aspect of the face and cheeks
     B. Headache
     C. Purulent nasal discharge
     D. Postnasal drip
     E. Congested, erythematous nasal mucosa
     F. Rarely, fever
 II. Treatment
     The treatment is surgical.
     A. Antral needle puncture may be performed to relieve symptoms and to obtain material for culture.
     B. A nasoantral window may be effective.
     C. A Caldwell-Luc procedure can be performed in more severe cases or those in whom the nasoantral window fails. With this operation, the maxillary sinus is opened, the mucosa is removed, and a nasoantral window is made.
III. Complications
     A. Persistent infection
     B. Oroantral fistulas

Chronic Ethmoiditis

Chronic ethmoiditis usually accompanies a long-standing infection of one of the other sinuses or prolonged nasal obstruction. There may be polypoid degeneration of the sinus mucosa presenting as obstructing nasal polyps.
  I. Signs and symptoms
     A. Purulent nasal discharge
     B. Dull headache between the eyes
     C. Nasal polyps or polypoid degeneration of the middle turbinates
 II. X-ray examination
     Opacification of the ethmoid sinus with loss of distinct bony septations can usually be seen on the submental vertex view.
III. Treatment
     Surgery is usually required. Either an intranasal or external ethmoidectomy can be performed and may be done in conjunction with surgery on one of the other sinuses. Drainage is established and any obstructing matter removed.
IV. Complications
     A. Orbital cellulitis/abscess

B. Meningitis
C. Cavernous sinus thrombosis

Chronic Sphenoiditis

The symptoms of chronic sphenoiditis vary greatly and are not common.
I. Signs and symptoms
   A. Dull, retro-orbital headache. The pain is usually throbbing but may not be a cardinal symptom of the disease.
   B. Purulent postnasal discharge. The discharge is usually thick, tenacious, and foul-smelling.
   C. Ocular symptoms. These include paralysis of the ocular muscles, fluctuating visual acuity, scotomas, diplopia, proptosis, and exophthalmos.
II. X-ray examination
   Radiographic changes show opacification of the sinus, with thickening of the mucosa.
III. Treatment
   A. Surgical drainage, accomplished by an intranasal approach, with removal of the anterior wall of the sphenoid sinus
   B. Intravenous antibiotics
   C. Decongestants
IV. Complications
   A. Meningitis
   B. Change in mental status. Long-standing chronic sphenoid sinusitis may cause loss of memory, depression, mental dullness, lack of concentration, and malaise. Such changes are likely due to diffuse cerebritis.
   C. Superior orbital fissure syndrome (paresis of cranial nerves III, IV, V, and VI)
   D. Retrobulbar neuritis
   E. Cavernous sinus thrombosis

UPPER RESPIRATORY INFECTIONS

Viral Upper Respiratory Infections

The classic "common cold" is the most frequent cause of infection in otolaryngology. A multitude of offending pathogens have been implicated including rhinovirus, influenza virus, parainfluenza virus, adenovirus, coxsackievirus, echovirus, reovirus, and respiratory syncytial virus.
I. Signs and symptoms
   A. Nasal stuffiness, usually with a gradual onset and lasting 3 to 7 days
   B. Malaise and fever

    C. Nasal discharge and watery rhinorrhea
    D. Edematous, erythematous nasal mucosa
    E. Sneezing and cough
    F. Anosmia
    G. Loss of taste
II. Treatment
    A. Hydration
    B. Analgesics
    C. Antihistamines: possibly helpful with excessive nasal secretions

Bacterial Upper Respiratory Infections

Bacterial upper respiratory infections (URI) are less common than viral URIs and may be accompanied by paranasal sinusitis. In children the offending organisms are usually *Hemophilus influenzae* or *Streptococcus pneumoniae*.[3] In adults, streptococci, staphylococci, and occasionally pneumococci are found.
 I. Signs and symptoms
    A. More persistent than viral infection
    B. Nasal obstruction
    C. Possibly associated with localized trauma or foreign body
    D. Tenacious, discolored, and malodorous nasal discharge
    E. Rarely, general body malaise
    F. Often associated with a preceding viral URI
    G. The oral mucosa may be more impressive than the nasal mucosa with a cobblestoned appearance of the posterior pharyngeal wall. Pus overlying the erythematous mucous membrane may be evident.
II. Treatment
    A. Amoxicillin in the pediatric age group
    B. Penicillin or amoxicillin in adults

TONSILLITIS

Tonsillitis is one of the infections that most commonly cause a patient to seek help from the family physician or emergency room physician.

Viral Tonsillitis

Viral tonsillitis is usually mild.
 I. Signs and symptoms
    A. Sore throat
    B. Dysphagia
    C. Fever

    D. Mildly enlarged tonsils without exudate

II. Treatment
    A. Fluids
    B. Aspirin or acetaminophen
    C. Bed rest when necessary

Beta-Streptococcal Tonsillitis

 I. Signs and symptoms
    A. Severe sore throat
    B. Dysphagia
    C. Fever
    D. Malaise
    E. Dehydration
    F. Enlarged tonsils with purulent exudate
    G. Beefy red, erythematous pharyngeal mucosa

II. Treatment
    A. Fluids: if the patient cannot take adequate fluids orally, hospitalization with intravenous fluids may be in order.
    B. Throat culture: 20% of population are carriers of this beta-Streptococcus in a normal state.
    C. Antibiotics: penicillin
    D. Bed rest when indicated

Mononucleosis

See also Chapter 8.

Severe tonsillitis is usually present with mononucleosis. Obtain a Monospot test to confirm the diagnosis of infectious mononucleosis. The treatment of choice for the overlying tonsillitis is penicillin. Avoid ampicillin because of the high incidence of skin rashes.

PERITONSILLAR ABSCESS/CELLULITIS

Peritonsillar abscess usually occurs in a patient who has not had previous problems with tonsillitis.

 I. Signs and symptoms
    A. Severe pain
    B. Fever
    C. Dysphagia
    D. Trismus
    E. "Hot potato" voice

    F. Erythema and enlargement of the offending tonsil
    G. Deviation of the tonsil toward the midline
    H. Fluctuance of the soft tissue between the superior pole of the tonsil and the soft palate
II. Treatment
    A. If trismus is severe, cocaine-soaked cotton pledgets are placed posteriorly under the middle turbinate.[4] This anesthetizes the sphenopalatine ganglion and breaks the trismus. In a patient with no trismus, the area can be anesthetized topically or injected with 1% xylocaine with 1:100,000 epinephrine.
    B. With adequate light and visualization, an 18 gauge needle may also be inserted into the fluctuant area of the tonsil with aspiration of the pus, avoiding an open incision.
    C. A 1 cm incision can also be made over the fluctuant area and a hemostat then inserted and spread to open the pocket of purulence.
    D. Pus is immediately sent for Gram stain and routine culture and sensitivity.
    E. Drainage of the abscess usually results in prompt relief of the severe pain.
    F. The patient is placed on oral antibiotics if able to tolerate oral medications.
    G. If the patient is unable to tolerate anything orally, he is hospitalized and placed on intravenous antibiotics. The most common cause for hospitalization in these patients is dehydration.
    H. Emergency tonsillectomy may be indicated. The infected tonsil or both tonsils may be removed. Bleeding is usually more troublesome in the acutely infected tonsil. A physician may also wait until the second serious infection before considering surgery. Approximately 20% of patients develop a second episode of peritonsillar abscess.[5] At that point both tonsils are usually removed.

LUDWIG'S ANGINA

    See also Chapter 7.
    Ludwig's angina is cellulitis of the floor of the mouth; 80% of the cases are of dental origin. Failure to recognize and treat this infection may result in progression of the disease and life-threatening complications.
  I. Signs and symptoms
    A. Tender cellulitis with edema in the floor of the mouth and induration and tenderness in the submandibular areas
    B. Dysphagia
    C. Odynophagia
    D. Inability to handle oral secretions
    E. Inability to close the mouth completely

F. Fever
G. Tongue displacement superiorly and posteriorly
H. Airway obstruction
II. Treatment
   A. Hospitalization
   B. Intravenous fluids
   C. Intravenous penicillin
   D. Close observation of the patient's respiratory status; management of the airway may include
      1. Nasopharyngeal airway
      2. Tracheostomy
      3. Routine intubation, which may be difficult in severe cases
   E. Surgical drainage may be necessary if there is no improvement on intravenous antibiotics. Because this is usually a phlegmon and not a frank abscess, drainage is reserved for refractory cases.

RETROPHARYNGEAL ABSCESS

See also Chapter 7.
Retropharyngeal abscess results from an accumulation of pus in the retropharyngeal space. This is an area bounded anteriorly by the posterior pharyngeal wall and posteriorly by the prevertebral fascia. It is primarily a disease of infants and young children.
  I. Signs and symptoms
   A. Neck pain
   B. Dysphagia
   C. Fever
   D. Loss of appetite
   E. Stiff neck
   F. Airway compromise
 II. Diagnosis
   Diagnosis may be difficult on clinical grounds alone. A fluctuant area in the oropharynx or hypopharynx may not be readily appreciated. The pain, dysphagia, and stiff neck alert the physician to the diagnosis, which can be confirmed with x-ray studies. A lateral neck x-ray film will show an increase in the AP soft tissue space anterior to the vertebrae that is 1.5 times the size of the adjacent vertebral body. Normally the adjacent soft tissue is less than one-third the diameter of the vertebral body.
III. Treatment
   A. Hospitalization
   B. Intravenous hydration
   C. Intravenous penicillin
   D. Airway observation. A tracheostomy set should be at the bedside in case of airway compromise.

    E. The retropharyngeal abscess is never drained in the emergency room. The patient is prepared for the operating room and the abscess incised and drained intraorally. If there is associated parapharyngeal space involvement, an external approach is planned. Antibiotics are continued throughout the postoperative period.

EPIGLOTTITIS

Epiglottitis most frequently occurs in children ages 3 to 6. In this age group the common offending organism is *Hemophilus influenzae* type B.[6] In the adult, epiglottitis is not as common and is thought to be of viral etiology. The basic symptom, airway compromise, is the same.

  I. Signs and symptoms
    A. Rapid onset of symptoms
    B. High fever
    C. "Hot potato" voice
    D. Inspiratory stridor
    E. Usually in a sitting position with the neck extended forward
    F. Severe sore throat
    G. Dysphagia
    H. Drooling
  II. Immediate evaluation
    A. Do not examine the mouth or attempt to visualize the epiglottis. Acute obstruction may result.
    B. Leave the parent with the child. If the child is sitting on the mother's lap and is comfortable, do not make an attempt to move him elsewhere for the sake of an examination.
    C. Do not be aggressive and push for a thorough examination. Perform those parts of the examination which may be necessary but do so in a controlled, soft-spoken voice.
    D. Do not lay the child down. Allow him to assume a comfortable sitting position.
    E. A lateral neck x-ray film may be obtained but *only* by portable x-ray technique in the emergency room. Under no circumstances should a child or adult be sent to the radiology department for an x-ray study, as there is the possibility of sudden, complete airway obstruction.
    F. Remember that this is an airway emergency, necessitating the presence of an anesthesiologist and an otolaryngologist. They must be called immediately, and the airway must be shared.
    G. The child is then transported to the operating room with an ambu bag and oxygen on the transporting table.
    H. If a child's airway is obstructed, do not attempt a tracheostomy in an uncontrolled situation. Ventilate with an ambu bag in standard fashion. Forceful ventilation can bypass even a large, swollen epiglottis.

III. Operative procedure
- A. A physician should stay in the operating room during the entire preoperative preparation.
- B. Bronchoscopy and tracheostomy sets should be available and set up in case there are problems establishing the airway.
- C. Light anesthesia may be administered, and the anesthesiologist plans an orotracheal intubation that can later be changed to nasotracheal intubation. No preoperative narcotics are given.
- D. In the rare event that the airway is lost, a bronchoscope is inserted. As soon as the patient is completely anesthetized, the bronchoscope can be removed and the nasotracheal tube placed.
- E. The otolaryngologist, emergency room physician, and anesthesiologist all examine the hypopharynx after intubation.
- F. Specimens for a blood culture and a culture of the tip of the epiglottis are taken.
- G. Intravenous antibiotics are started immediately. Ampicillin and chloramphenicol are instituted until 24 hour culture and sensitivity reports are available. Chloramphenicol is given initially because of the increasing resistance of *Hemophilus influenzae* to ampicillin. One drug can be discontinued after sensitivities have been determined.

IV. Postoperative care
- A. The patient is placed in the intensive care unit and sedated as necessary to secure the nasotracheal tube. The most common complication during this part of the treatment is accidental extubation.
- B. Antibiotic therapy is continued for a full 7 to 10 day course. After 48 to 72 hours, when the tube is removed, antibiotics may be changed to an oral route of administration.
- C. Extubation can usually be accomplished in 48 to 72 hours. The best way to ensure that the airway is healthy is to return the child to the operating room for an examination under anesthesia. Another helpful hint is the development of an air leak around the tube.
- D. If extubation cannot be accomplished after 72 hours, a tracheostomy is considered.

LARYNGOTRACHEAL BRONCHITIS (CROUP)

See also Chapter 8.

Croup is viral infection of the upper airway. It is usually caused by influenzae or parainfluenzae viruses.[7] Cases usually occur in clusters during the spring and fall and are primarily found in children ages 1 to 3 years.

I. Clinical features
- A. Low grade or moderate fever
- B. Barking, seal-like cough
- C. Inspiratory stridor

    D. Hoarseness

    E. Expiratory rhonchi

    F. Usually worse at night

    G. URI prodrome of several days' duration

II. Diagnosis

    Diagnosis is based on the above findings and radiographic changes. On x-ray films there is usually significant glottic and subglottic edema such that the subglottic airway is narrowed in an inverted funnel shape. This gives the telltale "steeple sign."

III. Treatment

    A. Humidification

    B. Racemic epinephrine may also be useful in viral croup. It may be given every hour during the acute phase with tapering as clinically necessary. This may avoid the need for more aggressive airway management.

    C. Rest

    D. Antibiotics are usually not given as this is a viral illness.

    E. Steroid use has proved beneficial in an inpatient population.[7]

    F. Mild cases may be treated on an outpatient basis. Patients with severe cases are hospitalized with monitoring of blood gases and careful attention paid to respiratory effort. Increasing respiratory and heart rates are signs of respiratory failure.

    G. In severe cases, intubation may be necessary. If the patient cannot be extubated between 48 to 72 hours, tracheostomy is considered.

BACTERIAL TRACHEITIS

See also Chapter 8.

Pediatric Tracheitis

Pediatric bacterial infection of the trachea is usually secondary to a foreign body. Foreign bodies in children are generally composed of vegetable matter and may cause a significant inflammatory response. With that, a purulent exudate results and may cause an ascending bacterial infection. There may be accompanying changes seen on the chest x-ray film. If possible, a bronchoscopic examination is performed with culture and sensitivity testing of the purulent matter. Great care is taken to look for foreign material and remove it.

Adult Tracheitis

Adult tracheitis may be associated with an acute pulmonary infection, most notably acute bronchitis. It may also be associated with tracheostomies where there is persistent contamination of the lower tracheobronchial tree without adequate clearing of mucus and other debris. In either case, it is very important to suction the purulent material and obtain a culture and sensitivity. The most common offending organisms are *Staphylococcus* and *Streptococcus*, and antibiotic therapy is directed toward these bacteria.

REFERENCES

1. Maresch MM: Paranasal sinuses from birth to late adolescence. Am J Dis Child 60:58, 1940
2. Evans FO, Sydnor JB, Moore WEC: Sinusitis of the maxillary antrum. N Engl J Med 293:735, 1975
3. Lepow M: Infections of the lower respiratory tract. p. 1251. In Bluestone CD, Stool SE (eds): Pediatric Otolaryngology. WB Saunders, Philadelphia, 1983
4. Kveton JF, Pillsbury HC: Breaking trismus to facilitate drainage of peritonsillar abscess. Laryngoscope 90:1892, 1980
5. Herbild O, Bonding O: Peritonsillar abscess. Arch Otolaryngol 107:540, 1981
6. Molteni RA: Epiglottitis: Incidence of extra-epiglottic infection; report of 72 cases and review of the literature. Pediatrics 58:526, 1976
7. Leipzig B, Oski FA, Cummings CW, et al: A prospective randomized study to determine the efficacy of steroids in the treatment of croup. J Pediatr 94:194, 1979

7

Face and Neck Infections

James Y. Suen
Bruce Leipzig _____

Major infections of the head and neck are not uncommon, and life-threatening complications may result if treatment is inadequate or delayed. Because the symptoms and signs associated with these infections are similar, the physician needs a thorough knowledge of them to diagnose the site of origin for proper treatment.

Infection and abscess formation spread through the head and neck by extension along fascial planes of least resistance. Because the fascia does not exclude one potential compartment from another, infection may spread across compartments and even into the mediastinum and thorax. This chapter outlines the symptoms and signs associated with infections of the face and neck and presents their differential diagnosis, treatment, and possible complications. This chapter is divided into several parts based on the anatomy of the face and neck (Fig. 7-1).

INFECTIONS OF THE ANTERIOR FACE

Skin/Scalp

Bacterial Infections

I. Folliculitis
   Predisposing factors include an unkempt beard, exposure to tar and mineral oils, and occlusive dressings, e.g., plaster.
   A. Signs and symptoms
      1. Usually little or no tenderness
      2. May be pruritic
      3. Scattered, discrete whitish pustules with adjacent erythema surrounding a hair follicle
      4. Common distribution: the male beard areas of the face
   B. Treatment
      1. Removal of the causative agent, e.g., tar or mineral oil
      2. Local hygiene (soap and water)
      3. Removal of hair follicle(s) if single or few

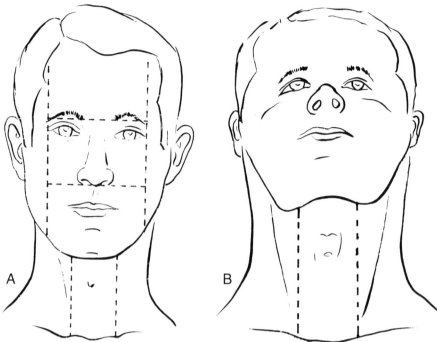

Fig. 7-1. (A) Face divided into anatomic regions. (B) Neck divided into anterior and lateral compartments.

       4. Topical antibacterial agents
       5. Systemic antibiotics—usually not necessary
II. Furuncle (boil) and carbuncle
    A furuncle is erythematous and indurated, and may have central ulceration and necrosis. A carbuncle is a group of furuncles organized into one lesion.
   A. Signs and symptoms
       1. Throbbing pain and exquisite tenderness
       2. Occasionally low-grade fever and malaise
       3. Common on the face, but most common where there are hair follicles and in areas subject to friction and sweating (nose, neck, face)
   B. Laboratory examination
      Swab of pustules or ulceration for Gram stain, culture, and antibiotic sensitivity studies
   C. Differential diagnosis
       1. Herpes simplex, necrotic type
       2. Foreign body
       3. Acne
   D. Treatment
       1. Simple furuncle

a) Remove hair, when this is the cause
b) Heat, moist when possible
c) Systemic antibiotics usually unnecessary unless the patient is immunosuppressed or has diabetes

2. Furuncle with surrounding cellulitis and fever, or carbuncle
a) Systemic antibiotics, e.g., oxacillin or erythromycin, for 1 week
b) Incision and drainage if abscess present

3. Recurrent furunculosis
a) All of the above plus daily application of antibacterial ointments
b) Underlying cause sought, e.g., diabetes
c) Surgical excision occasionally necessary

E. Complications
1. Carbuncle formation
2. Facial cellulitis
3. Abscess formation
4. Sepsis

III. Infected epidermal cyst

Most epidermal cysts arise from occluded pilosebaceous follicles, although some occur along embryonic closure lines.[1] They are usually asymptomatic until they become infected.

A. Signs and symptoms
1. Redness, pain, and swelling of overlying skin
2. Edematous punctum of pilosebaceous gland often visible
3. Often associated with acne vulgaris

B. Treatment
1. Antibiotics effective against *Staphylococcus aureus*
2. Hot compresses
3. Incision and drainage necessary if abscess occurs
4. Cyst excised after inflammation subsides

IV. Impetigo

Impetigo usually occurs in preschool children and young adults in crowded living conditions as a result of poor hygiene and neglected minor trauma.

A. Signs and symptoms
1. Pruritic lesions commonly present for days prior to the patient seeking medical treatment
2. Clusters of crusted lesions from oozing serum
3. Lesions discrete and scattered or may become large and confluent; many caused by autoinoculation with the patient's fingernails
4. Regional lymphadenopathy

B. Laboratory examination
1. Gram stain of lesions reveals gram-positive cocci in chains or clusters.
2. Culture reveals group A streptococci predominating in a mixed culture.

C. Differential diagnosis
   1. In an early stage of vesicles, impetigo may simulate varicella and herpes simplex.
   2. Tinea corporis; shows mycelia on smear
D. Treatment
   1. Local cleansing with soap and water
   2. Antibiotic ointment containing neomycin or bacitracin for mild cases
   3. Penicillin for 10 days for severe cases or those in which beta-streptococci group A are cultured
   4. Erythromycin if patient cannot take penicillin
   5. *Note:* Lesion is infectious and the patient's sheets and clothing should be isolated during the period of the infection.
V. Cellulitis
   Predisposing factors include malnutrition, stasis dermatitis, lymphedema, nephrotic edema, and other immune malformations.
   A. Signs and symptoms
      1. Pain and tenderness of involved skin
      2. Abrupt onset of 2 to 5 days
      3. Systemic symptoms of acute illness with headaches, chills, fever, and weakness
      4. Toxic appearance of patient, with fever
      5. Enlarging margin of swollen skin, bright red in appearance
      6. Indurated skin with peau d'orange appearance
      7. Area of infection warm to touch
      8. Diffuse involvement over a large area of skin surface
   B. Laboratory examination
      1. Elevated white blood cell (WBC) count
      2. Blood cultures
   C. Types of cellulitis and differential diagnosis
      1. Erysipelas: Form of cellulitis caused by beta-streptococci
      2. *Hemophilus influenzae* cellulitis (Fig. 7-2)
         a) Rapid onset of signs and symptoms
         b) Slightly purple hue to skin
      3. Secondary cellulitis
         a) Often associated with predisposing infection, e.g., furuncle, carbuncle
         b) Culture the precipitating lesion.
      4. Angioneurotic edema: usually presents without erythema or fever
      5. Brown recluse spider bite: presents as cellulitis with central necrosis
   D. Treatment depends on the type of cellulitis
      1. Penicillin for erysipelas
      2. Amoxicillin for *Hemophilus influenzae* infection

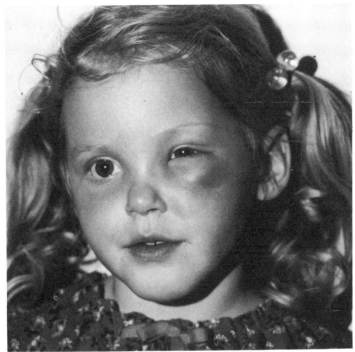

Fig. 7-2. Child with *H. influenzae* cellulitis resulting in periorbital edema and erythema.

3. Antistaphylococcal agent if furuncle or carbuncle suspected as etiologic factor
   E. Prognosis
      1. With high dose antibiotics most cases resolve.
      2. If untreated, it may go on to abscess formation.
VI. Abscess
   A. Signs and symptoms
      1. Pain
      2. Persistent or spiking fever
      3. Redness, swelling, and tenderness
      4. Often firm and tense overlying skin
      5. Sometimes edema of skin
      6. Abscess may "point" and drain spontaneously if untreated.
      7. Usually there is a precipitating infection, e.g., furuncle or dental infection.
   B. Laboratory examination
      1. Abscess is aspirated with a needle to confirm the diagnosis and to obtain material for culture and sensitivity.
      2. Elevated WBC count
   C. Treatment

1. Incision and drainage
    a) Usually performed with local anesthesia, though it is difficult to obtain good local anesthesia because the acidity of the environment partially neutralizes the analgesic effect. Topical freezing agents may also be used to provide anesthesia.
    b) If the abscess is large, insertion of a Penrose drain, gauze packing, or a gauze wick prevents the incision from closing before the infection has cleared.
    c) If packing or a wick is inserted, it must be replaced often to prevent it from serving as a focus of continuing infection.
2. Intravenous antibiotics

Viral Infections

I. Herpes simplex
    Most commonly the primary infection occurs between the ages of 1 and 5 and in young adults. Herpes can recur after exposure to ultraviolet radiation, sunlight, or trauma such as dermabrasion, and in those who are immunosuppressed. Asymptomatic carriers do exist and may transmit the disease. The incubation period is 2 to 20 days.
    A. Signs and symptoms
        1. Burning, itching, and pain in the lesions
        2. Possible constitutional symptoms of headache and fever
        3. Vesicles arranged in clusters on an erythematous base (herpetiform)
        4. In primary infections lesions occur most commonly on the lips but are also seen frequently in the mouth; when lesions recur, they distribute anywhere on the face and lips but only rarely on the mucous membranes.
        5. Regional adenopathy is common in primary herpes but uncommon in recurrent herpes.
    B. Laboratory examination
        1. Tzanck cell test preparation[2]: Unroof the blister top carefully and gently scrape the base of the lesion on the slide. Allow it to air-dry. Toluidine blue staining reveals a typical pattern, with multinucleated giant cells, faceted nuclei, and "ground glass" chromatin.
        2. Virus culture is more specific but less readily available.
    C. Differential diagnosis
        1. Impetigo
        2. Eczema
        3. Syphilitic chancres
        4. Herpes zoster
    D. Treatment

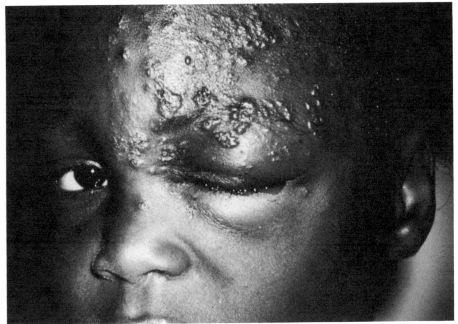

Fig. 7-3. Herpes zoster.

1. Acyclovir: topical 5% ointment is applied every 3 hours for 7 days at onset of symptoms and signs—very effective if applied early but not effective after full-blown lesions appear.[3]
   2. Topical antibiotics are sometimes helpful.
   3. Creams containing dimethylsulfoxide (DMSO) do not prevent relapses.
   E. Complications
   1. Relapse of herpes simplex infections is common.
   2. Lesions occasionally result in scarring.
II. Herpes zoster
   A. Signs and symptoms
   1. Pain and paresthesias, with itching, tingling, and burning in the involved dermatome preceding the eruption by several days. Pain can be severe and usually is present for the duration of active lesions.
   2. Constitutional symptoms are rare.
   3. Papules occur in 24 hours and change to vesicles and bullae. After 4 days pustules with crusting occur. New lesions may continue to appear for up to 1 week.
   4. Distribution of these vesicles and bullae is along a dermatome and is therefore usually unilateral (Fig. 7-3). In approximately 20% of herpes zoster cases, lesions occur in the cervical region.

B. Laboratory examination
   Virus culture
C. Differential diagnosis
   It is especially important to differentiate between herpes simplex and herpes zoster.
D. Treatment
   1. Corticosteroids are controversial but may be of some benefit (especially in herpes zoster of ophthalmic area). Use prednisone 60 mg daily in divided doses for 1 week with decreasing doses for the next 3 weeks.
   2. Pain medications are given.
   3. With severe pain, amitripyline (Elavil) 50 to 100 mg at bedtime and fluphenazine (Prolixin) 1 mg q8h may be helpful.
   4. Calamine lotion is applied to dry the lesions.
   5. Acyclovir is being tested for intravenous use and may be effective.
E. Complications
   1. Postherpetic neuralgia occurs in 30% of patients over 40 years of age and can last for years. Ophthalmic herpes zoster is especially associated with this postinfectious pain.
   2. Ophthalmic complications and loss of vision may occur.
   3. If the ear is involved, facial nerve paralysis (herpes zoster oticus) may occur.

Upper One-Third of the Face

Infections in the forehead region are very unusual except as manifestations of frontal sinus disease. If there is tenderness, erythema, swelling, and/or pain over the frontal sinuses, these sinuses must be suspected and evaluated for infection (see Ch. 6).

Middle One-Third of the Face

Periorbital Area

I. Etiology
   Sinus infections are the most common cause of periorbital infections. The ethmoid sinuses are the most common site, followed by the frontal and maxillary sinuses. Periorbital edema may occur in the absence of orbital infections and may represent inflammation or trauma of the cheek, nose, or forehead.
II. Radiographic evaluations
   A. Sinus radiographs are helpful for the detection of sinus infections that may result in periorbital disease.

    B. Ultrasound can help detect orbital abscesses and localize them.

    C. Computed tomography (CT scan) is helpful for diagnosing and localizing orbital abscesses.

III. Periorbital edema

    A. Signs and symptoms

       1. Eyelid swelling

       2. Absence of proptosis or other eye abnormalities

    B. Treatment

       Treat underlying disease.

IV. Orbital cellulitis

    A. Signs and symptoms

       1. Swelling and erythema of lids, chemosis (conjunctival edema), pain, and tenderness

       2. Possible mild to moderate proptosis

       3. Possible restriction of eye movement and visual impairment.

    B. Treatment

       1. Intravenous antibiotics usually produce improvement within 24 hours; if no improvement or if the disease is progressing, an abscess is probably present.

       2. Sinus disease, if present, is treated.

V. Subperiosteal abscess

    A. Signs and symptoms

       1. Swelling and erythema of lids, chemosis, pain, and tenderness, but usually progressive and more severe than in orbital cellulitis

       2. Possible restriction of eye movements, proptosis, and visual impairment

       3. Possible lateral displacement of eye due to presence of pus between lamina papyracea (medial orbital wall) and periorbita

    B. Treatment

       1. Incision and drainage above medial canthal ligament combined with external ethmoidectomy

       2. Intravenous antibiotics

VI. Orbital abscess

    A. Signs and symptoms

       1. Swelling and erythema of lids, chemosis, pain, and tenderness, but usually progressive and more severe than in orbital cellulitis

       2. Restriction of eye movement, proptosis, and visual impairment

    B. Treatment

       1. Incision and drainage via upper lid or lower lid depending on site of abscess

       2. Intravenous antibiotics

       3. Sinus disease treated if present

VII. Cavernous sinus thrombosis

    A. Signs and symptoms

       1. Patient very ill

      2. Retrobulbar pain
      3. Proptosis and ophthalmoplegia
      4. Decreasing vision
      5. Papilledema
      6. Possible meningitis
    B. Treatment
      1. Intensive antibiotics
      2. Anticoagulation drug therapy
      3. Surgical decompression of any involved sinuses
VIII. Complications
    A. Loss of vision
    B. Cellulitis and abscess, sometimes leading to cavernous sinus thrombosis
    C. Osteomyelitis
    D. Intracranial infections

Nose

  I. External skin infections
    See infections of the skin of the anterior face, above.
 II. Dermoid cysts
    Dermoid cysts are located on the dorsum of the nose and may produce progressive swelling if infected (Fig. 7-4). They may be associated with an intracranial sinus tract.[4]
III. Vestibular skin infections
    A. The most common vestibular "lesion" of the nose results from the common cold (see Ch. 6).
    B. Superficial folliculitis
      1. Signs and symptoms
        a) Irritation and erythema as seen in other superficial folliculitis (see section on folliculitis, under Skin/Scalp, above).
        b) Erythema with possible pustule formation around the hair follicles of the anterior nares
      2. Laboratory examination
        Culture and sensitivity testing may be performed, but usually the diagnosis is clear and treatment for a staphylococcal infection is appropriate.
      3. Treatment
        a) Topical antibiotic ointment
        b) Systemic antistaphylococcal antibiotic therapy, e.g., dicloxacillin
        c) Erythromycin in the penicillin-sensitive patient
      4. Complications
        a) Cellulitis and abscess formation

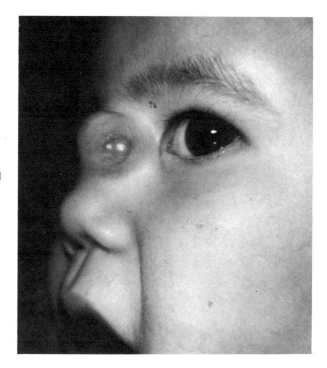

Fig. 7-4. Child with dermoid cyst of the nasal dorsum.

      b) Chrondritis of the overlying nasal cartilages

IV. Septal abscess

    The most common etiology of septal abscess is nasal trauma with a septal hematoma that becomes infected. A septal hematoma may be overlooked and confused with edema, so a careful examination is essential.

    A. Signs and symptoms

        1. Nasal obstruction

        2. Pain and tenderness upon palpation and movement of the nasal septum

        3. Bulging of septum, usually bilateral

    B. Differential diagnosis

        1. Deviated nasal septum

        2. Septal hematoma

    C. Laboratory examination

        The only test necessary is aspiration of the nasal septum with a large needle to check for pus or blood.

    D. Treatment

        1. Incision and drainage of septum

        2. Gauze packing in the abscess cavity

        3. Systemic antibiotics; penicillin preferred

        4. Erythromycin or cephazolin in the penicillin-sensitive patient

     5. Gauze packing, changed daily for 2 or 3 days; after that, packing usually not necessary
  E. Complications
     1. Dissolution of septal cartilage with consequent septal collapse and internal nasal obstruction
     2. "Saddle nose" deformity
V. Rhinitis (see Ch. 6)
VI. Foreign bodies (see Ch. 13)

Cheek

  I. Acne
    Cystic acne with secondary infection occasionally presents as a facial infection. This is treated similarly to a furuncle.
 II. Cellulitis
    See Skin/Scalp infections, above.
III. Maxillary sinusitis
    These may present as swelling and redness over the cheeks (see Ch. 6).
IV. Dental infections
    These may present as swelling, tenderness, and redness over the lower cheek areas. The teeth should be checked (see Ch. 15).

Lower One-Third of the Face

Lips

  I. Trauma with secondary infection
 II. Herpes simplex (see above)
III. Angioneurotic edema[5] (see also Ch. 8)
  A. Etiology
    1. Allergy—physical and food
    2. Drug reaction
    3. Infection
  B. Signs and symptoms
    1. Hives (urticaria)
    2. Partial or entire lip swelling
    3. New lesions continuing to appear
    4. Lesions may itch.
    5. Individual lesions may be transient.
    6. Constitutional symptoms include hoarseness, stridor, and dyspnea.
  C. Treatment
    1. Search for and removal of the etiologic factor

2. Systemic antihistamines, e.g., diphenhydramine hydrochloride (Benadryl) 25 to 50 mg i.m. or p.o. every 4 hours
3. Systemic corticosteroids if rapidly progressive and unresponsive to Benadryl; dexamethasone 8 mg i.m. or i.v. initially, then 4 mg every 6 hours until controlled

IV. Stevens-Johnson syndrome[6]
  A. Etiology
    1. Drug reactions
    2. Viral infections
    3. Bacterial infections
    4. *Mycoplasma* infections
    5. Deep mycoses
    6. Malignant neoplasms
  B. Signs and symptoms
    1. Rapid onset
    2. A form of erythema multiforme, with lesions of the mucosal surfaces of the mouth, lips, eyes, and genitalia
    3. Constitutional symptoms of high fever, headaches, and prostration
  C. Treatment
    1. Must be initiated promptly
    2. Corticosteroids, such as dexamethasone 8 mg i.v. or i.m. initially, then 4 mg every 6 hours
    3. Immediate ophthalmic consultation to treat conjunctival lesions because of possible blindness ensuing
    4. Parenteral alimentation

Chin

The chin rarely has a significant infection. If present, it is usually related to a skin infection (see previous section).

INFECTIONS OF THE LATERAL FACE: PAROTITIS

Parotitis[7] is usually related to obstruction of the parotid duct or results from bacteria ascending the duct from the mouth; alternatively, it is a viral infection.
  I. Signs and symptoms
    A. Pain upon eating or constant pain
    B. Swelling, redness, and tenderness
    C. Possible trismus
 II. Differential diagnosis
    A. Acute suppurative parotitis
    B. Mumps
    C. Lymphadenitis

    D. Obstructive parotitis due to duct stricture or to a stone

    E. Tumor with necrosis or inflammatory reaction

III. Acute suppurative parotitis

    A. Diagnosis

       1. Predisposing factors: debilitation or dehydration (frequently postoperative)

       2. Tender, swollen gland

       3. Possible purulent drainage from parotid duct

       4. Usually *Staphylococcus* infection

       5. May result in fistulas or abscess

       6. Rarely, fluctuance due to the dense fascia surrounding the gland

    B. Treatment

       1. Antibiotics to treat *Staphylococcus aureus*, e.g., dicloxacillin sodium

       2. Hydration or fluid replacement

       3. If abscess suspected, aspirate for pus; if present, incise and drain in the operating room

    C. Complications

       1. Chronic parotitis

       2. Abscess formation

       3. Facial nerve paralysis

       4. Fistulas

       5. Lateral pharyngeal space extension

IV. Mumps

    A. Diagnosis

       1. Viral etiology

       2. Usually in children 4 to 6 years of age but may occur in adults

       3. Usually bilateral

       4. Diffuse swelling and tenderness

       5. Low grade fever

       6. Sometimes orchitis in adult men

    B. Treatment

       1. Symptomatic treatment only

       2. Antibiotics not indicated

    C. Complications

       1. Orchitis with sterility, usually in adults

       2. Unilateral sensorineural hearing loss, usually in children

V. Lymphadenitis

    A. Diagnosis

       1. Usually it is a more localized infection than parotitis.

       2. Often multiple nodes are enlarged.

    B. Treatment

       1. Try to find a specific infection, e.g., cat scratch fever, then treat appropriately.

    2. If no obvious etiology, treat with antibiotics, e.g., penicillin, erythromycin, or a cephalosporin.

  C. Complication: abscess

VI. Obstructive parotitis

  A. Diagnosis

    1. Secondary to duct stricture or calculus

    2. Swelling and pain frequently related to eating

    3. No pus from duct

    4. Usually no organisms involved

    5. Sialogram, if no active infection, usually demonstrates a stricture or calculus.

  B. Treatment

    1. Attempt to alleviate obstruction by dilating the duct or breaking up calculus with dilator probe.

    2. Antibiotics are given.

    3. May require parotidectomy if condition does not resolve.

  C. Complications

    1. Chronic sialoadenitis

    2. Fistulas

    3. Abscesses

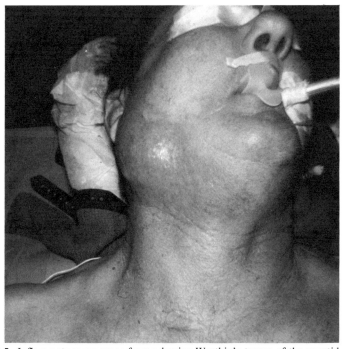

Fig. 7-5. Inflammatory response from a benign Warthin's tumor of the parotid gland.

VII. Tumor with necrosis or inflammatory reaction
    A. Diagnosis
        1. Some tumors of the parotid have cystic degeneration with a secondary inflammatory response (Fig. 7-5).
        2. There is usually a history of a mass present with inflammation occurring later.
    B. Treatment
        1. Antibiotics
        2. Aspiration if cyst or abscess suspected
        3. Incision and drainage only if necessary
        4. Resection of tumor and parotid when inflammation improves
    C. Complications
        1. Recurrent tumor
        2. Fistulas

INFECTIONS OF THE ANTERIOR NECK

Infections of the anterior neck are uncommon but are fairly easy to diagnose. The large majority of infections seen in the anterior neck are associated with one of several disorders.[7]
    I. Ludwig's angina
   II. Infected thyroglossal duct cyst
  III. Cervical lymphadenitis
  IV. Thyroiditis
   V. Anaplastic carcinoma of the thyroid

Ludwig's Angina

    I. Etiology
        A. Most commonly from dental infections (80%)
        B. Lacerations and infections in the floor of the mouth
        C. Salivary calculi
        D. Fractures of the mandible
   II. Signs and symptoms
        A. Swelling, induration, and erythema in the submental and submandibular areas and the floor of the mouth
        B. Displacement of the tongue superiorly and posteriorly
        C. Tongue immobility, dysphagia, and excess salivation
        D. Pain in the floor of the mouth
        E. Voice changes secondary to tongue immobility
        F. Fever
        G. Mild to moderate respiratory distress
  III. Diagnosis

A. Dental evaluation

B. Dental occlusive view x-ray films to identify possible calcifications (stone formation) in the submandibular ducts

C. Mandible radiographs, if indicated by history and physical examination, to identify fractures or recent dental trauma

D. Culture and sensitivity of any draining or aspirated purulent substance. Gram stain may give important immediate information to guide antibiotic therapy.

IV. Treatment

A. Antibiotics: penicillin or cephazolin intravenously

B. Surgical exploration and drainage

1. Surgery is indicated if there is no marked improvement within 24 hours or if symptoms progress to abscess formation or respiratory obstruction.

2. An intraoral approach is indicated if an abscess appears to "point" in the floor of the mouth.

3. An external approach through the submental area is preferred. This approach must go through the mylohyoid muscle, as the infection involves areas both above and below the muscle.

C. Tracheotomy possibly necessary if respiratory obstruction is present

V. Complications

A. Tongue retrusion sometimes progressive, leading to airway compromise

B. Deep neck cellulitis and abscess if the mylohyoid muscle is penetrated by infection

C. Extension of infection into mediastinum and thorax

D. Aspiration of purulent material into the lungs

Infected Thyroglossal Duct Cyst

I. Signs and symptoms

A. History of a soft mass in the midline of the neck near the hyoid bone which moves with swallowing (Fig. 7-6)

B. Recent swelling, erythema, and tenderness of the mass and anterior neck

C. Pain especially upon swallowing

II. Diagnosis

A. Culture and sensitivity of any draining or aspirated purulent material. Gram stain may give important immediate information to guide antibiotic therapy. The cysts are usually sterile, and the inflammation may be secondary to rupture of the cyst.

B. If the thyroid gland is not easily palpable, it is prudent to obtain a thyroid scan prior to surgical intervention.

III. Treatment

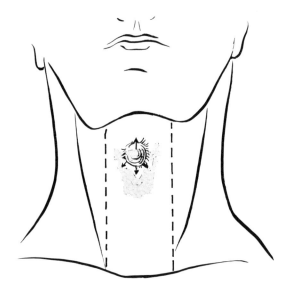

Fig. 7-6. Typical location of a thyroglossal duct cyst.

   A. Antibiotics. Penicillin is the drug of choice. If it is a severe infection, intravenous antibiotics are indicated.
   B. Incision and drainage if there is not marked improvement within 24 hours or if symptoms progress to abscess formation or respiratory obstruction.
   C. When the acute infection has resolved, definitive resection of the thyroglossal duct cyst is required.
IV. Complications
   A. Deep neck cellulitis and abscess
   B. Respiratory obstruction
   C. Aspiration

Cervical Lymphadenitis

  I. Signs and symptoms
   A. Tenderness and enlargement of one or more lymph nodes in the submental area
   B. Most cases associated with either viral upper respiratory tract infections or bacterial infections of the teeth or tonsils
 II. Diagnosis
   A. Obtain history regarding recent upper respiratory tract infection or dental problems.
   B. Examine lower face and oral cavity for infection.

    C. If the cause of the lymphadenitis remains unknown and the lymphadenitis does not respond to treatment, a tuberculin skin test, cultures of the throat, and serology for infectious mononucleosis, toxoplasmosis, and cytomegalovirus infection can be performed.

    D. If the lymph node is large and persistent, biopsy is indicated.

III. Treatment

    A. Systemic antibiotics such as penicillin or a cephazolin

    B. If no response to antibiotic treatment then perhaps excisional biopsy.

IV. Complications

    Deep neck cellulitis and abscess

Thyroiditis

Hashimoto's autoimmune thyroiditis is the most common form of thyroiditis. Acute suppurative thyroiditis is very rare.

  I. Signs and symptoms

    A. Acute enlargement of part or all of the thyroid

    B. Occasionally, tenderness and pain radiating to the ear

    C. Rarely, symptoms of tracheal compression

      1. Cough

      2. Dysphagia

      3. Respiratory difficulty

    D. Rarely, transient hyperthyroidism symptoms with subacute thyroiditis

    E. Late in the disease process there may be signs of hypothyroidism, e.g., listlessness, changes in voice, and changes in swallowing.

 II. Diagnosis

    A. Serum T_4 and T_3 levels may be increased, decreased, or normal.

    B. Thyroid-stimulating hormone (TSH) may be low, high, or normal.

    C. Erythrocyte sedimentation rate (ESR) increased

    D. Antithyroid antibodies

    E. Laryngeal examination for vocal cord paralysis

    F. Needle biopsy of thyroid gland

III. Treatment

    A. Aspirin, an ice collar, and propylthiouracil are effective for subacute thyroiditis. Rarely, steroids and x-ray therapy are required.

    B. Thyroid hormone suppression for Hashimoto's thyroiditis is applied in the absence of symptoms of tracheal compression.

    C. Surgical resection or tracheotomy is rarely indicated, except in the presence of compression symptoms.

IV. Late complications

    A. Hypothyroidism

    B. Respiratory obstruction

    C. Dysphagia

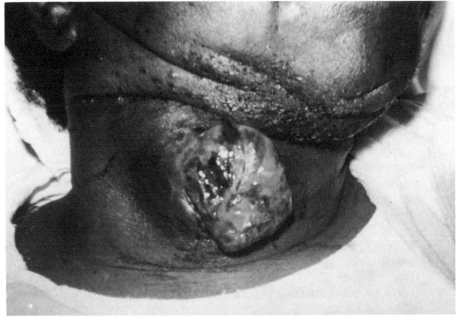

Fig. 7-7. Fungating anaplastic carcinoma of the thyroid gland.

Anaplastic Carcinoma of the Thyroid

I. Signs and symptoms
  A. Usually seen in patients over 60 years of age and most often in women
  B. Rapid, diffuse glandular enlargement with overlying inflammatory changes (Fig. 7-7)
  C. Vocal cord paralysis, hoarseness
  D. Dysphagia
  E. Respiratory distress
  F. Fixation to muscles, skin, trachea, and esophagus
II. Diagnosis
  A. Laryngeal examination for vocal cord function
  B. Thyroid scan shows decreased uptake
  C. CT scan to determine extent of tumor invasion
  D. Needle biopsy
  E. Open biopsy if needle biopsy negative
III. Treatment
  A. Tracheotomy is done for airway obstruction; it is usually difficult and performed through the tumor.
  B. Surgical resection is often not possible due to the extensive disease that is usually present.

   C. Radiation therapy combined with chemotherapy may be helpful for palliation.
IV. Complications
   A. Respiratory obstruction due to bilateral recurrent laryngeal nerve involvement or tracheal compression may occur.
   B. Survival is usually less than 1 year.

INFECTIONS OF THE LATERAL NECK

Infections of the lateral neck can be very difficult to diagnose because only a few of them originate in the neck. It is important to do a complete head and neck examination in order not to miss the primary lesion, e.g., a carcinoma of the pharynx with necrosis or a neck metastasis. The following disorders account for the majority of lateral neck infections.[8]
  I. Submandibular gland sialoadenitis
 II. Cervical lymphadenitis
III. Deep neck infections
IV. Infected branchial cleft cyst
 V. Neck metastasis with necrosis
VI. Lymphoma

Submandibular Gland Sialoadenitis

  I. Signs and symptoms
   A. Pain and swelling in the submandibular triangle
   B. Symptoms exacerbated by eating
   C. Erythema surrounding the opening of the submandibular duct in the floor of the mouth
   D. Turbid or purulent drainage from the submandibular duct
   E. Submandibular gland tender to external or bimanual palpation
   F. Stones in the duct or gland, often palpable, the most common source of submandibular gland infection
 II. Diagnosis
   A. Culture and sensitivity studies of ductal secretions for both aerobic and anaerobic infections. A Gram-stained smear of any pus is appropriate.
   B. Dental occlusive view radiographs to look for calculi in the floor of mouth. Approximately 80% of calculi can be seen radiographically with proper x-ray studies.
III. Treatment
   A. Vigorous hydration is used.
   B. Antibiotics: Penicillin is the drug of choice. If systemic signs of infection are present, intravenous penicillin is preferred.

C. Surgical intervention is necessary if there are signs of progression or abscess formation.
D. Surgical treatment includes incision and drainage of the submandibular space from an external approach. If the gland is abscessed, gland excision is appropriate after the infection resolves.

IV. Complications
A. Deep neck cellulitis and abscess formation
B. Hypoglossal nerve paralysis

Cervical Lymphadenitis

See Infections of the Anterior Neck above.

Deep Neck Infections

Deep neck space infections can occur in any of the triangles of the neck as the result of spread of infection from a primary site. Identification of the primary source of infection must be made at the time of treatment of deep space infection.

I. Signs and symptoms
A. Swelling is most often centered just inferior to the angle of the mandible (Fig. 7-8)
B. Trismus. It may be difficult to examine the mouth because of limitation in opening the mouth from the inflammatory process involving the muscles of mastication.
C. Bulging of the posterior or lateral pharyngeal wall. Once the mouth is open, a mass or a bulging can often be seen and palpated.
D. Drooling
E. Dysphagia
F. "Hot potato" voice
G. Posturing of the neck to the contralateral side
H. Tongue retrusion with submandibular space involvement, which may be progressive owing to limitation of the swelling by the mylohyoid muscle sling. This may progress to the point of airway compromise.
I. Fluctuance of the neck is almost never noted owing to the deep location of these abscesses.

II. Diagnosis
A. Soft tissue radiographs are helpful for diagnosing a retropharyngeal abscess. The normal thickness of the postpharyngeal soft tissue overlying C5 as seen on a lateral neck x-ray film should measure no greater than 1.5 times the anteroposterior (AP) width of C5 in a child less than 1 year of age, no greater than one-half the AP width of C5 in a child

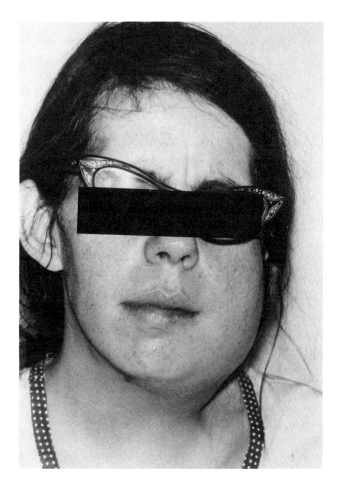

Fig. 7-8. Deep neck abscess.

between 1 and 6 years of age, and no greater than one-third the AP width of C5 from the age of 6 into adulthood.[9]
  B. Needle aspiration is performed for culture and sensitivity (aerobes and anaerobes) if an abscess is suspected.
  C. If incision and drainage are required, consider a biopsy of wall of abscess.
  D. CT scan is used to localized abscess formation.
III. Treatment
  A. Any patient with progressing deep neck infection must be hospitalized for treatment.
  B. Rehydration is accomplished with intravenous fluids.
  C. High dose intravenous antibiotics are started. If no cultures and sensitivities are available, the antibiotics suitable for suspected organisms include high dose penicillin and/or one of the synthetic drugs active against *Staphylococcus aureus* and pathogenic streptococci. Anaer-

obic bacteria are also commonly present in abscess formations of the head and neck but are usually sensitive to penicillin. A Gram-stained smear of any pus may reveal important pathogenic information early.
  D. If there is no improvement of symptoms within 24 to 48 hours, or if signs of progression or abscess formation have developed, surgical treatment is mandatory.
  E. Deep neck infections must be recognized early and followed with aggressive medical and surgical treatment in order to prevent life-threatening complications. Conservative observation may be more radical when a greater threat to life is involved with such complications as septic embolism and carotid artery erosion. In such instances, surgery is the more conservative approach.
IV. Complications
  A. Extension of infection, especially into the mediastinum and chest. This mandates immediate surgical intervention.
  B. Spread along the carotid sheath anteriorly or the prevertebral fascia posteriorly
  C. Retrograde thrombophlebitis in the internal jugular vein with resulting septicemia
  D. Erosion of major vessels such as the carotid or internal jugular vein
  E. Respiratory obstruction
  F. Aspiration pneumonia
  G. Occasionally, paralysis of any of the major nerve trunks adjacent to the carotid sheath

Infected Branchial Cleft Cyst

  I. Signs and symptoms
  A. May or may not have history of a previous asymptomatic neck mass
  B. Rapid enlargement of a mass in the upper one-half of the neck
  C. Tenderness, pain, and occasionally fever
  D. If ruptured, cellulitis with brawny edema of the skin of the neck
 II. Diagnosis
  A. Culture and sensitivity of any draining or aspirated purulent material. Gram stain may give important immediate information to guide antibiotic therapy; however, the abscess may be sterile.
  B. CT scan
  C. Diagnosis may not be evident until surgical excision is performed, revealing epithelial elements.
III. Treatment
  A. Antibiotics: Penicillin is the drug of choice. If there are signs of systemic infection or rupture, intravenous antibiotics are necessary.

B. Surgery is indicated if there is no improvement within 24 to 48 hours, symptoms progress to abscess formation, or respiratory obstruction occurs.
   C. When the acute infection is resolved, definitive resection of the branchial cleft cyst is required.
IV. Complications
   A. Deep neck cellulitis and abscess
   B. Respiratory obstruction
   C. Aspiration
   D. Recurrent neck abscesses

Cervical Node Metastasis with Necrosis

Central necrosis is common in metastatic neck nodes which are large. The necrotic nodes can simulate an infection and must be considered in the differential diagnosis of a neck infection. The nodes are usually sterile unless secondary infection occurs after incision and drainage or spontaneous rupture.
   I. Signs and symptoms
      A. Slowly enlarging neck mass which gradually becomes tender
      B. Frequently attached to the skin with overlying erythema
      C. May be cystic and fluctuant just beneath the skin
      D. May be fixed to adjacent structures
      E. May have symptoms from the primary tumor, e.g., hoarseness or dysphagia
      F. Occasionally, involvement of adjacent cranial nerves with paralysis of nerves IX, X, XI, or XII or Horner's syndrome
      G. Usually do not respond to antibiotics
  II. Diagnosis
      A. Thorough head and neck examination
      B. Biopsy of any suspicious lesions
      C. Biopsy of wall of cystic mass after incision and drainage
      D. Culture and sensitivity of any drainage
 III. Treatment
      A. Thoroughly evaluate for the primary cancer, then treat appropriately.
      B. Antibiotics are not usually helpful. Clindamycin may be useful if there is secondary infection.
      C. Definitive treatment is usually surgery and/or irradiation.
 IV. Complications
      A. Cranial nerve paralysis
      B. Uncontrolled neck disease
      C. Carotid artery rupture
      D. Death

Lymphoma

I. Signs and symptoms
   A. May be asymptomatic mass(es)
   B. May be tender, painful mass(es)
   C. May be multiple nodes of variable sizes
   D. May involve extranodal sites such as the tonsils
II. Diagnosis
   A. Careful head and neck examination
   B. Excisional or incisional biopsy of mass
III. Treatment
   A. Systemic evaluation
   B. Irradiation versus chemotherapy
IV. Complications
   A. Systemic disease
   B. Death

REFERENCES

1. Caro WA, Bronstein BF: Tumors of the skin. p. 1540. In Moschella SL, Hurley JH (eds): Dermatology. 2nd Ed. Saunders, Philadelphia, 1985
2. Solomon AR, Rasmussen JE, Varani J, Pierson CL: The Tzanck smear in the diagnosis of cutaneous herpes simplex. JAMA 251:633, 1984
3. Corey L, Nahmias AJ, Guinan ME, et al: A trial of topical acyclovir in genital herpes simplex virus infections. N Engl J Med 306:1318, 1982
4. Sessions RB: Nasal dermal sinuses—new concepts and explanations. Laryngoscope, suppl. 29, 92:1, 1982
5. Fitzpatrick TB, Polano MK, Suurmond D: Color Atlas and Synopsis of Clinical Dermatology. p. 118. McGraw-Hill, New York, 1983
6. Petersdorf RG, Adams RD, Braunwald E, et al (eds): Harrison's Principles of Internal Medicine. 9th Ed. p. 70. McGraw-Hill, New York, 1982
7. Leipzig B, Obert P: Parotid gland swelling. J Fam Pract 9:1085, 1979
8. Rabuzzi DD, Johnson JT: Diagnosis and Management of Deep Neck Infections. Self-Instructional Package. Committee on Continuing Education in Otolaryngology, American Academy of Ophthalmology and Otolaryngology, 1976
9. Lusted LB, Keats TE: Atlas of Roentgenographic Measurement. p. 28. Medical Publishers, Chicago, 1978

8

Airway Obstruction

Robert W. Seibert
Stephen J. Wetmore

AIRWAY OBSTRUCTION IN INFANTS AND CHILDREN

In infants and children the upper airway, extending from the nares to the carina, differs from adults in the following ways:

1. The airway has a smaller diameter. In the upper airway of infants and children the cross-sectional area of the airway decreases proportionately to a much greater degree than in larger individuals. For this reason lesions that might produce minimal or no symptoms in an adult's airway might cause severe or life-threatening problems in an infant. The laryngeal subglottic airway has the smallest cross-sectional area of the upper airway. The subglottic mucosal and submucosal tissue is more loosely attached to its framework, thereby allowing edema fluid to readily accumulate here and obstruct the airway.[1]

2. Infants, especially newborns, are obligate nasal breathers; therefore obstruction of the nasal airway results in severe symptoms and may be life-threatening.

3. The larynx is located higher in the neck than in adults, with the inferior border located at the level of the third or fourth cervical vertebra. The epiglottis is long, narrow, and curled upon itself, often with loosely attached, redundant aryepiglottic folds which tend to prolapse into the airway lumen on inspiration.

The terminology used here includes the following:

Snoring (stertorous breathing): indicates nasopharyngeal or oropharyngeal airway obstruction

Stridor: a hard, high-pitched respiratory sound such as the inspiratory sound often heard in acute laryngeal obstruction

Biphasic stridor: inspiratory and expiratory stridor, usually heard with lesions involving the trachea

Hoarseness: roughened, often harsh quality to the voice or cry, indicative of a lesion of the true vocal cord

Croup: presence of a brassy, metallic cough. Only lesions in the subglottic larynx produce a croupy cough.

Wheeze: whistling sound made in breathing. Primarily heard with bronchial obstruction.

"Hot potato voice": resonance of the voice changed to a muffled, thickened, but not hoarse quality. Points to a lesion involving the oropharynx (tonsils, soft palate, posterior pharyngeal wall) or hypopharynx, base of tongue, vallecula, or epiglottis.

Drooling: excessive salivation which runs out the mouth

Dysphagia: difficulty swallowing

Odynophagia: painful swallowing or sore throat

There are certain general principles involved in treating children with airway obstruction.

1. The first sign of hypoxia due to an obstructed upper airway may be agitation.

2. Supplemental oxygen is given and the cause of the upper airway obstruction sought and treated appropriately.

3. Because of the danger of respiratory arrest in an already hypoxic patient, sedatives or analgesics are contraindicated because they may further depress respiration.

ANATOMIC SITES AND SPECIFIC CAUSES

Nose

Choanal Atresia

Choanal atresia is persistence of the bony (usually) or membranous plate at the posterior choanae. If bilateral, it results in complete obstruction of the nasal airway and is life-threatening because of the neonate's obligate nasal breathing.

I. Signs and symptoms
   A. Severe respiratory distress with retractions and cyanosis that improves when the infant cries, at which time mouth breathing occurs. May do fairly well except when feeding.
   B. Bilateral mucoid nasal discharge
   C. Inability to pass catheters through the nose
   D. Diagnosis may be confirmed by x-ray films of the nose with contrast material (metrizamide) placed in each side.

II. Treatment
   A. Establish an airway. A McGovern nipple may be made by cutting the end off a baby bottle nipple and taping the remainder of it in the baby's mouth. This forces the baby to breathe through the mouth and also serves as a route for oral feedings (Fig. 8-1).[2]
   B. Refer to an otolaryngologist for a more permanent airway. The procedure of choice is transnasal resection of the atresia plate and stenting of the opening with tubes that also maintain the airway.[3] Later a transpalatal procedure is done if necessary.

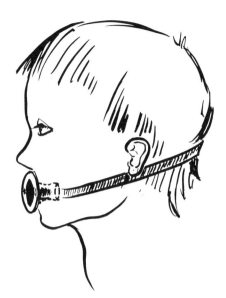

Fig. 8-1. McGovern nipple in a child with choanal atresia.

Nasal Encephalocele

The nasal encephalocele is a congenital defect consisting of brain tissue herniating into the nose through a defect of the skull base, usually the cribriform plate.

I. Signs and symptoms
   A. Suspect if hypertelorism is present.
   B. Some patients have recurrent meningitis.
   C. Soft tissue mass may be difficult to detect on sinus x-ray films; do computed tomography (CT scan) for definitive diagnosis.

II. Treatment
   Combined otolaryngologic and neurosurgical approach is often required.[4]

Nasopharynx

Adenoidal Hypertrophy

I. Signs and symptoms
   A. Enlargement of the adenoid pad is very common in children over 1 year of age.
   B. Symptoms are mouth breathing when awake and snoring when asleep.
   C. Occasionally obstructive sleep apnea occurs, resulting in hypoxemia and hypercarbia; pulmonary hypertension may result, leading to right heart failure (cor pulmonale).
   D. Tonsillar hypertrophy is commonly found as well.

    E. Lateral nasopharyngeal x-ray films show size of the adenoid pad relative to nasopharyngeal dimensions and airway.

II. Treatment

    Adenoidectomy

Nasopharyngeal Angiofibroma

The nasopharyngeal angiofibroma is a benign but often locally aggressive neoplasm of adolescent boys that arises from the nasopharyngeal roof. Its occurrence in female subjects is extremely rare.[5]

  I. Signs and symptoms

    Symptoms are gradually increasing nasal airway obstruction and nosebleeds. The tumor is highly vascular, and epistaxis may be severe.

  II. Diagnosis

    Diagnosis is made by the characteristic clinical presentation and radiographic studies

 III. Treatment

    Treatment is surgical excision, often preceded by embolization via angiography to decrease blood supply to the tumor.

Oral Cavity

Robin's Sequence (Robin Anomalad, Pierre Robin Syndrome)

  I. Signs and symptoms

    A. This congenital facial anomaly consists in a small retruded mandible that causes the tongue to fall back into the pharynx, producing airway obstruction and feeding difficulties.

    B. A posterior U-shaped cleft palate occurs in 40% of cases.[6]

  II. Treatment

    A. Airway and feedings are managed by keeping the infant in a prone position with head down so that the tongue falls forward.

    B. Feedings via orogastric tube or gastrostomy may be necessary.

    C. In severe cases tracheotomy may be necessary to protect the airway.

    D. A palatal feeding prosthesis may be of benefit in the patient with a cleft palate.

    E. Surgical procedures to attach the tongue anteriorly (glossopexy) have had limited success.[7]

Ludwig's Angina

Ludwig's angina consists of cellulitis of the sublingual and submandibular spaces, usually from a dental infection.

I. Signs and symptoms
   Swelling above the mylohyoid muscle pushes the tongue upward and posteriorly, obstructing the airway.[7]
II. Laboratory examination
   Aspiration is done to obtain specimens for a Gram stain and culture for offending organisms.
III. Treatment
   A. Intensive intravenous antimicrobial therapy (penicillin G or clindamycin) is begun and the airway supported as needed.
   B. Occasionally tracheotomy is required.

Macroglossia

The causes of an enlarged tongue (macroglossia) are many (cretinism, storage diseases, lymphangioma, Beckwith syndrome). Airway obstruction is rarely acute.

Oropharynx

Tonsillar Hypertrophy

Chronic partial airway obstruction secondary to noninfected, hypertrophic tonsils and adenoids is very common in children (see adenoidal hypertrophy). Emergency removal of the tonsils and adenoids is not indicated except in a case of severe obstructive sleep apnea, especially associated with acute cardiac decompensation (cor pulmonale) or life-threatening cardiac arrhythmias.

Hypopharynx

Retropharyngeal Abscess

See also Chapter 7.
Retropharyngeal lymph nodes lie in two vertical chains on either side of the midline in the retropharyngeal space and receive lymph drainage primarily from the nasopharynx and the eustachian tube. They are most prominent in children less than 4 years of age, and therefore infection of the retropharyngeal space is most likely to occur in young children. Retropharyngeal adenitis–cellulitis may progress to abscess formation. The cause is usually nasopharyngitis or trauma, especially a perforating foreign body. Most common organisms are group A *Streptococcus, Staphylococcus aureus,* and aerobic and anaerobic pharyngeal microorganisms.[7]
I. Signs and symptoms

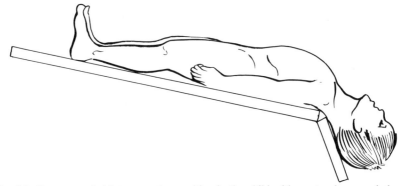

Fig. 8-2. Recommended intraoperative position in the child with a retropharyngeal abscess.

   A. Fever
   B. Dysphagia, drooling
   C. Stiff neck, possibly opisthotonos
   D. Stridor and airway obstruction if swelling is severe enough to encroach
      on the airway
  II. Diagnostic studies
   A. Lateral x-ray film of the neck shows widening of the retropharyngeal
      space. Must rule out artificial widening produced by malposition of
      infant on x-ray table.
   B. Fluoroscopy resolves questionable cases. Air density in retrophar-
      yngeal space indicates infection by gas-producing organisms or com-
      munication with pharynx or esophagus.
 III. Treatment
   A. This disease is considered a life-threatening emergency. Incision and
      drainage of the abscess via a transoral route with control of the airway
      via endotracheal tube is the treatment of choice. A tracheotomy may
      be necessary if the airway obstruction is severe. Patient is positioned
      supine with head and upper body in a dependent position (Rose and
      Trendelenburg position) (Fig. 8-2). Abscess may be unilateral due to
      a median raphe of the retropharyngeal space. Aspiration with needle
      and syringe is done first to obtain exudate for Gram stain plus culture
      and sensitivity as well as to locate the abscess.
   B. Antimicrobials: Penicillin G, 5 million to 10 million units per day via
      intravenous route. If *S. aureus* is suspected on Gram stain, use naf-
      cillin. In penicillin-allergic patient, clindamycin is drug of choice be-
      cause of its antimicrobial spectrum including anaerobic organisms.
 IV. Complications
      Spontaneous rupture of the abscess may result in serious, possibly fatal,
   complications.
   A. Anteriorly—into airway with asphyxiation or aspiration pneumonia.

B. Posteriorly—into spine with subluxation of cervical vertebrae due to dissolution of ligaments or osteomyelitis
C. Laterally—into lateral pharyngeal space with thrombosis or erosion of great vessels
D. Inferiorly—into mediastinum with possible extension to diaphragm

Supraglottic Larynx

Laryngomalacia

Laryngomalacia is flaccidity of supraglottic structures in infants with collapse of the aryepiglottic folds and arytenoids into the airway lumen on inspiration. It accounts for 60% of laryngeal obstruction in infants.[8]
  I. Signs and symptoms
      A. Onset of fluttering inspiratory stridor appears at birth or shortly thereafter.
      B. Stridor increases when infant is agitated and decreases in the prone position or when neck is hyperextended.
      C. May have retractions, but severe respiratory distress is very uncommon.
      D. Feeding is usually normal.
 II. Diagnosis
      A. Characteristic clinical picture noted above
      B. Videofluoroscopy shows redundant, wavy aryepiglottic folds.
      C. Definitive diagnosis is by direct laryngoscopy or flexible fiberoptic laryngoscopy in an awake infant. Collapse of the supraglottic larynx seen on inspiration.
      D. May coexist with other congenital obstructive lesions such as subglottic stenosis, which should be ruled out.
III. Treatment
      Because this condition is almost always mild and resolves gradually with time, parental reassurance is all that is usually needed.

Epiglottitis

Epiglottitis is severe infection of the supraglottic larynx. It is associated with high morbidity and mortality in children due to a rapid and severe upper airway obstruction unless promptly diagnosed and managed correctly.
  I. Etiology
      Hemophilus influenzae type B is the most common organism (50 to 75% of cases). *Streptococcus pneumoniae* and beta-hemolytic *Streptoccocus* have been cultured but are much less common.
 II. Signs and symptoms

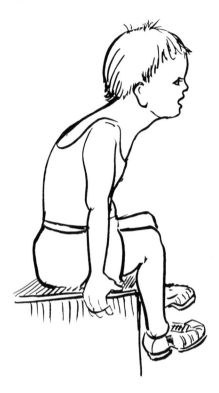

Fig. 8-3. Usual position of the child presenting with epiglottitis.

A. Sudden onset and rapid progression of inspiratory stridor occurring over hours. The most common age is 3 to 6 years, but it may occur at any age.
B. Inspiratory stridor: coarse fluttering sound
C. Patients maintain "sniffing position" (Fig. 8-3).
D. High fever
E. Ill appearing ("toxic")
F. "Hot potato" voice
G. Severe dysphagia, drooling
H. Epiglottis appears enlarged to several times normal size and is inflamed with bright cherry red to purplish beefy red color. *No attempt is made to examine the throat of any child with suspected epiglottitis unless the examiner is prepared to intubate the trachea immediately.* Any manipulation of the airway or even change in position may precipitate complete airway obstruction.
III. Radiography. Lateral x-ray of the neck shows enlarged epiglottis ("thumb sign"). X-ray studies are usually unnecessary. If done, patient is accompanied to the radiology department by someone capable of intubating the trachea. Films are taken with patient in the upright position.
IV. Treatment

A. Airway: As soon as the diagnosis is made an artificial airway is established in *all* children.[9]
   1. Because an airway is required for 48 to 72 hours, endotracheal intubation, preferably nasotracheal intubation, is desirable so long as constant monitoring is available. Otherwise tracheotomy may be used to provide the temporary airway.
   2. If a mildly symptomatic patient needs to be transported to another facility, the airway is established prior to transport and is maintained by experienced personnel constantly in attendance unless the transport time is extremely short.
B. Antimicrobials
   1. Obtain swab of epiglottis for culture and sensitivity and blood cultures at the time of intubation.
   2. Administer ampicillin, 150 to 200 mg/kg/24 hours intravenously.
   3. Because of the possibility of resistant strains of *H. influenzae* type B, also begin chloramphenicol, 100 mg/kg/24 hours, until culture and sensitivity results are known.[10]
C. Steroids
   Steroids may be used just prior to extubation to avoid postintubation subglottic edema. They have no role in the treatment of the acute infection.

Allergic Supraglottic Edema (Angioneurotic Edema)

See section on Airway Obstruction in Adults.

Glottic Larynx

Glottic Atresia/Stenosis

Glottic atresia requires immediate tracheotomy in the delivery room. Most cases are diagnosed at autopsy. Glottic stenosis is secondary to an anterior web, frequently associated with subglottic stenosis.

Bilateral Vocal Cord Paralysis

I. Signs and symptoms
   A. Moderate to severe inspiratory stridor
   B. Hoarse cry sometimes, but usually strong
II. Diagnosis
   A. Frequently associated with central nervous system (CNS) anomalies such as hydrocephalus or Arnold-Chiari malformation.

B. Fluoroscopy of the larynx may be strongly suggestive, but definitive diagnosis is made by endoscopy.
III. Treatment
   A. Treatment of the CNS anomaly, e.g., by shunting the hydrocephalus, may improve the airway.
   B. In idiopathic bilateral vocal cord paralysis the conditon may spontaneously improve.
   C. Tracheotomy may be necessary if airway symptoms are prominent.

Unilateral Vocal Cord Paralysis

I. Signs and symptoms
   A. Weak, hoarse cry
   B. Feeding problems with possible aspiration
   C. Airway obstruction not usually prominent unless associated with superimposed stress, e.g., upper respiratory infection.
II. Diagnosis
   A. Diagnosis is made by endoscopy
   B. Commonly associated with cardiovascular disease but may be due to vagal nerve injury anywhere from the brain to the chest
III. Treatment
   Vocal cord paralysis in the neonate or child does not usually require treatment, although the underlying cause may need to be treated.

Laryngeal Trauma

See Chapter 3.

Subglottic Larynx

Congenital Subglottic Stenosis

Congenital subglottic stenosis is caused by malformation of the cricoid cartilage or, more commonly, soft tissue stenosis.
I. Signs and symptoms
   The degree of airway distress depends on the severity of the stenosis, ranging from asymptomatic stridor and croup associated only with infections to severe stridor at rest.
II. Diagnosis

A. Soft tissue lateral x-ray film of airway
B. CT scan to define cricoid lesion (optional)
C. Endoscopy. Subglottic airway of normal newborn should admit a 3.5 mm endotracheal tube

III. Treatment

May require tracheotomy. The subglottic larynx enlarges as the patient grows so that decannulation usually is possible by age 1 to 2 years. Direct surgical approach to stenosis is usually deferred.

Acquired Subglottic Stenosis

Acquired subglottic stenosis, an extremely difficult management problem, is commonly seen after long-term endotracheal intubation and may follow laryngeal fracture. This condition is much more difficult to treat than the congenital type and is more variable in severity and in its response to treatment.

I. Symptoms are inspiratory stridor and croupy cough, sometimes progressing to severe obstruction.
II. Diagnosis is by radiographic studies and endoscopy.
III. Treatment
A. In infants, particularly premature ones, with prolonged endotracheal intubation, cricoid split procedure may avoid tracheotomy.[11]
B. Fresh strictures may respond to dilatations and steroid injections.
C. Firm cicatricial strictures or long segments require open laryngotracheoplasty with reconstructive surgical techniques and stenting.[12]
D. Tracheotomy
1. Temporary tracheotomy is needed in most cases.
2. Permanent tracheotomy may be needed if other treatments fail.

Laryngotracheobronchitis (Croup)

Laryngotracheobronchitis (LTB) is a common disease during winter and spring in children 2 years old and younger. The cause is a virus, especially influenza, parainfluenza, and respiratory syncytial viruses.

I. Signs and symptoms
A. Upper respiratory tract prodrome progresses over days with hoarseness, croupy cough, mild to moderate inspiratory stridor, low grade or no fever.
B. Severe respiratory distress is rare.
C. No dysphagia or drooling is seen.
D. Patient may be in any body position.
II. Diagnosis
A. Diagnosis is made by clinical presentation.

    B. Lateral x-ray film of neck shows subglottic narrowing.

    C. Endoscopy usually is not necessary to make diagnosis.

III. Treatment

    A. Majority of patients may be treated at home with humidification, general supportive care. With severe stridor and obstruction, especially patient retaining CO_2, hospitalization is necessary. In the severe case, dexamethasone 0.3 mg/kg initially and repeated in 2 hours may be beneficial in improving the airway and avoiding intubation.[13] Racemic epinephrine by updraft or intermittent positive pressure breathing may also reduce subglottic edema.

    B. Artificial airway: Endotracheal tube or tracheotomy is required in small percentage of cases. Airway is needed for 1 to 2 weeks in some cases.

Trachea

Congenital Tracheal Anomalies

Except for extremely rare and severe tracheal anomalies (agenesis, atresia), congenital problems causing tracheal airway obstruction are unlikely to present as acute emergencies. Congenital anomalies of the great vessels ("vascular ring") may produce stridor, wheezing, and cough due to impingement on the trachea and larger bronchi. Dysphagia and feeding difficulties may occur with concomitant esophageal compression. Collapse of the tracheal lumen on inspiration (tracheal malacia) is a diagnosis of exclusion, as it may be secondary to vascular compression or tracheoesophageal fistula.

Bacterial (Suppurative) Tracheitis

Severe bacterial infection of the trachea causes airway obstruction due to copious purulent secretions. It may follow a bout of viral LTB or occur without preexisting viral infection. The organism is almost always *Staphylococcus aureus*.[14]

    I. Signs and symptoms

        Inspiratory stridor, croupy cough, fever progressing over 12 to 24 hours—more slowly than with epiglottitis, faster than with LTB

   II. Diagnosis

    A. Made by characteristic clinical symptomatology in association with signs of bacterial infection, e.g., leukocytosis with left shift.

    B. Lateral x-ray film of neck shows narrowed tracheal air column with irregular configuration due to exudate.

III. Treatment

A. Airway: Most patients require endotracheal intubation or tracheotomy.
B. Antistaphylococcal antibiotics are given intravenously.

AIRWAY OBSTRUCTION IN ADULTS

A large variety of diseases can cause airway obstruction. A useful way of approaching the patient with airway distress is to consider the most likely group of causes in his age group in light of the findings of the history and physical examination. A distinctly different group of causes is usually found in children than in adults, although there is some overlap, e.g., trauma. In this part of the chapter the causes of airway obstruction in adults are discussed, and specific techniques for managing airway obstruction are presented.

DIFFERENTIAL DIAGNOSIS

  I. General: There are many diseases, e.g., nasal polyps, which can result in some airway obstruction but are not life-threatening. Only those diseases or situations which may result in complete airway obstruction are discussed.
 II. Trauma
     A. Facial fractures
     B. Laryngotracheal trauma
     C. Postintubation trauma
III. Infection
     A. Ludwig's angina
     B. Infectious mononucleosis
     C. Diphtheria
     D. Epiglottitis
     E. Tetanus
     F. Retropharyngeal abscess
 IV. Neoplasms
     A. Carcinoma of the laryngopharynx
     B. Carcinoma of the trachea or adjacent structures (thyroid, esophagus)
  V. Foreign body
 VI. Miscellaneous
     A. Anaphylactic reaction
     B. Angioneurotic edema
     C. Bilateral vocal cord paralysis
     D. Cricoarytenoid arthritis

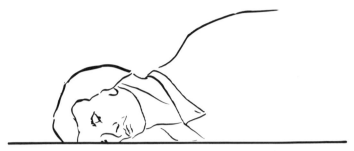

Fig. 8-4. Positioning the patient on his side without a pillow under his head allows secretions to flow from the mouth by gravity and often avoids oropharyngeal obstruction by the tongue.

TRAUMA

Severe Facial Fractures

  I. A displaced comminuted fracture of the anterior mandible can result in loss of support of the tongue, causing posterior tongue displacement and oropharyngeal airway obstruction.
 II. Often a midface fracture is also present, making insertion of a nasopharyngeal airway difficult.
III. If the patient can be positioned on his side (Fig. 8-4) or prone, temporary improvement of the airway may be obtained.
 IV. If the patient cannot be repositioned, temporary airway relief may be obtained by manually holding the anterior mandible forward (Fig. 8-5).

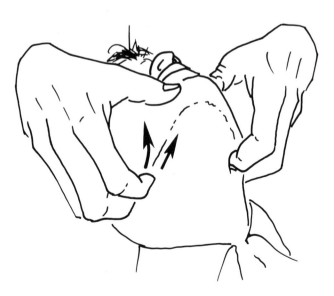

Fig. 8-5. Jaw thrust maneuver. Lift the angle of the mandible away from the cervical spine.

V. Orotracheal intubation may be difficult owing to bleeding and tongue edema.
VI. Definitive airway support is achieved by either tracheotomy or cricothyroidotomy.

Laryngotracheal Trauma

Either blunt or penetrating trauma to the neck can result in airway obstruction. See Chapter 3 for discussion of this problem.

Trauma from Instrumentation

I. Previous prolonged intubation with endotracheal tubes may cause injury to the trachea or subglottis, resulting in a stenosis. The obstruction may not be obvious until as short as 1 week or as long as months after extubation. Anytime a patient is seen for airway obstruction and the cause is not obvious, a history of previous instrumentation should be ascertained.
II. Previous tracheotomy, especially if the patient required a ventilator, may result in stenosis and obstruction several weeks to months later and should be considered as a cause of obstruction.
III. Signs and symptoms
   A. Subglottic area: stridor, dyspnea, weak voice
   B. Trachea: dyspnea, prolonged inspiration and expiration
IV. Diagnosis
   A. History of previous instrumentation
   B. Above signs on physical examination
   C. Larynx and trachea tomograms
   D. Laryngoscopy and bronchoscopy
V. Treatment
   A. If there is a very localized and thin segment of stenosis, repeated dilatations may be effective.
   B. Steroid injections into the stenosis are occasionally helpful.
   C. For subglottic stenosis in adults that does not respond to either of the above treatments, a hyoid interposition or a prolonged stent insertion may be necessary.
   D. For tracheal stenosis that does not respond to the above, a tracheal resection may be necessary.
   E. A tracheotomy may be necessary if the obstruction is severe and other measures are not helpful.

INFECTIONS

Ludwig's Angina (Floor of Mouth Cellulitis)

A nasopharyngeal airway or a tracheotomy may be necessary. See Chapter 6 for a discussion of this problem.

Infectious Mononucleosis

  I. Etiology
     Epstein-Barr virus
 II. Signs and symptoms
     A. Sore throat, dysphagia, and marked general malaise usually occur.
     B. Airway impairment may be seen with marked enlargement of the palatine tonsils.
     C. The tonsils may meet in the midline of the oropharynx.
     D. The tonsils are edematous and covered by a gray-white exudate.
     E. Concomitant bacterial tonsillitis may be present.
     F. Cervical lymph nodes are invariably enlarged and tender bilaterally.
     G. A fever of up to 103° to 105°F may occur.
     H. Petechiae located at the junction of the hard and soft palate are highly suggestive, although not pathognomonic.
     I. Splenomegaly occurs in 50% of cases.
III. Laboratory examination
     A. Monospot test may need repeating in 1 to 2 weeks if negative initially.
     B. Heterophil antibody test: Only 60% of patients with infectious mononucleosis have a positive test within the first 2 weeks after onset of the illness; 90% have a positive test 1 month after onset.[15]
     C. White blood cell (WBC) count
        1. Greater than 50% lymphocytes
        2. Greater than 10% atypical lymphocytes
     D. Culture and sensitivity of tonsils
 IV. Treatment
     A. If airway impairment is imminent, hospitalize and give corticosteroids.
     B. Treat for possible bacterial tonsillitis if airway impairment is imminent or culture shows bacteria.
        1. Penicillin is drug of choice.
        2. Avoid ampicillin because of the high incidence of rash reported when used for this disease.
     C. Nasopharyngeal airway may be needed while patient responds to the above measures.
     D. Only rarely is tracheotomy or emergency tonsillectomy needed.

Diphtheria

  I. Etiology
     A. *Corynebacterium diphtheriae*, a gram-positive rod, causes the pharyngeal inflammation, and its toxin produces myocarditis and peripheral neuritis.
     B. It is transmitted by droplet exposure from active cases or carriers via the upper respiratory tract.

II. Signs and symptoms
  A. Early in the course of this disease a thin, easily wiped off membrane forms over the pharynx and tonsils.
  B. As the disease progresses the membrane thickens, becomes gray to black, and is firmly attached to the mucosa, resulting in mucosal bleeding when attempts are made to remove it.
  C. Marked spread of the membrane can take place throughout the mouth, pharynx, and larynx, resulting in airway obstruction.
    1. Stridor, thick speech, and foul breath occur.
    2. Pharynx becomes red and edematous.
    3. Cervical lymph nodes enlarge from secondary infection.
    4. Membrane extends, on rare occasions, into the tracheobronchial tree.
  D. Complications may be due to diphtheria toxin.
    1. Myocarditis
    2. Paralysis of soft palate and pharyngeal wall
    3. Other cranial neuropathies, mainly of motor nerves initially
    4. Peripheral neuropathies occur late in the course of the disease.
III. Diagnostic tests
  A. Smear for *C. diphtheriae* organism
  B. Culture and sensitivity: Loeffler's medium shows growth in 12 hours if patient has not been taking antibiotics.
IV. Prevention, treatment, prognosis
  A. Diphtheria toxoid as part of childhood immunizations provides protection from diphtheria.
  B. If diphtheria is suspected, antitoxin is administered immediately; the antitoxin is effective only against the toxin in the bloodstream, not against intracellular toxin.
  C. Consider endotracheal intubation or tracheotomy for patients with impaired upper airway.
  D. Humidify the upper airway.
  E. Antibiotics may not affect the course of the illness.
  F. Penicillin or erythromycin is used to treat diphtheria carriers.
  G. Overall death rate in United States in treated patients is 10%.[16]

Epiglottitis

I. Etiology
  A. Although *Hemophilus influenza* type B can cause epiglottitis in the adult, the incidence of this organism in adults is much lower than in children with epiglottitis.[17]
  B. *Streptococcus pneumoniae*, beta-hemolytic streptococci, and *Staphylococcus aureus*, as well as viruses, may cause this disease in adults.[18]
II. Signs and symptoms

A. Sore throat, dysphagia, and odynophagia
B. Low grade fever
C. Stridor may not be an initial symptom in adults as it is almost invariably in children.
D. Indirect laryngoscopy reveals an erythematous, edematous epiglottis.
E. If untreated, stridor and airway compromise may ensue.

III. Treatment
A. Intravenous antibiotic: amoxicillin unless allergic to penicillin
B. Intravenous corticosteroids, e.g., dexamethasone
C. Close monitoring of airway
  1. If edema progresses, consider intubation or tracheotomy.
  2. Because the adult's airway is much larger than the child's, airway support is less frequently required in the adult with epiglottitis.[19]

Tetanus

I. Etiology
A. *Clostridium tetani*, an obligate anaerobe and a large, motile, spore-forming gram-positive bacillus, causes tetanus.
B. Most of the manifestations of the disease are due to an exotoxin.

II. Signs and symptoms
A. Spasm of the muscles of mastication results in trismus (lockjaw).
B. Sustained contraction of the facial muscles produces the distorted grin of risus sardonicus.
C. Dysphagia from spasm of pharyngeal muscles
D. Stiff neck
E. Pain from muscle spasm
F. Apprehension, profuse sweating, low grade fever, and tachycardia
G. Hyperactive tendon reflexes with clonus
H. Convulsions sometimes precipitated by minor stimuli
I. Possibly, laryngospasm

III. Differential diagnosis[20]
A. Peritonsillar abscess often causes trismus.
B. Phenothiazine reaction may result in extrapyramidal tract findings of facial dystonia.
C. Meningitis produces a stiff neck but not the other manifestations of tetanus.
D. Strychnine poisoning may produce hyperexcitability of muscles as in tetanus, except that the muscles are relaxed between seizures in strychnine intoxication.

IV. Treatment
A. Tracheotomy: Patient is given a muscle relaxant and intubated by the anesthesiologist prior to tracheotomy to avoid laryngospasm with complete airway obstruction.

B. Patient is kept in a quiet, darkened room and managed with central nervous system (CNS) sedatives.

C. Antitoxin: human tetanus immune globulin cannot neutralize toxin already in the CNS.

D. Immunization: see Chapter 2.

E. Surgical wound débridement may be necessary.

F. Intravenous penicillin is recommended, but antibiotics may not influence the progression of the disease.

NEOPLASMS

I. Etiology

Most neoplasms of the upper aerodigestive tract that cause airway obstruction are squamous cell carcinomas and are located in the laryngopharynx, trachea, or adjacent structures, e.g., thyroid or esophagus.

II. Signs and symptoms

A. Most of these patients have had symptoms of hoarseness, shortness of breath, dysphagia, odynophagia, or hemoptysis for weeks to months prior to their symptoms of respiratory distress.

B. On the other hand, neoplasms of the subglottic larynx, trachea, and proximal bronchi may be asymptomatic except for progressive shortness of breath and stridor.

C. Examination of the pharynx and larynx usually reveals an ulcerated and/or exophytic mass.

D. Cancer of the larynx may have fixation of a vocal cord with a lesion.

E. Chest and neck x-ray films usually detect an obstructing mass in the trachea or bronchi.

III. Treatment

A. Tracheotomy is usually necessary to secure the airway in most cases of obstructing head and neck cancer.

B. If an intrinsic carcinoma of the larynx is suspected, direct laryngoscopy under general anesthesia and debulking of the tumor with the CO_2 laser may avoid tracheotomy until the time of laryngectomy.

C. If an intrinsic tumor in the distal trachea or proximal bronchi is suspected, rigid bronchoscopy and debulking of the tumor may be necessary because proximal tracheotomy may not be able to bypass the area of obstruction. The CO_2 or neodynium-YAG lasers are useful tools for debulking the lesion.

FOREIGN BODIES

See Chapter 6.

MISCELLANEOUS CAUSES

Anaphylactic Reaction

I. Etiology
   A. Anaphylaxis is an immediate hypersensitivity reaction to a foreign antigen, usually mediated by immunoglobulin E (IgE) antibody.
   B. The two most common antigens to cause anaphylaxis are penicillin and Hymenoptera stings.[21]
II. Signs and symptoms
   A. Rapid onset of symptoms, usually within 30 minutes of exposure to the antigen
   B. Initial symptoms are often a tingling of the face or mouth followed by a feeling of generalized warmth.
   C. A sense of fullness or tightness in the throat and chest often follows.
   D. The patient may complain of a feeling of impending doom.
   E. Pruritis of the eyes, nasal congestion, hoarseness, coughing, sneezing, chest pain, and generalized sweating often ensue.
   F. Lip, tongue, pharyngeal, and laryngeal edema and inspiratory stridor may be seen.
   G. If airway impairment is moderately severe, cyanosis of the lips, face, and nailbeds will be present.
   H. Wheezes, rales, and rhonchi often can be heard.
   I. Hypotension, distant heart sounds, and arrhythmias are seen with severe reactions.
   J. Respiratory arrest, coma, and death are rare but certainly can occur.
III. Differential diagnosis
   A. Vasovagal collapse is the main condition to differentiate from anaphylaxis.
      1. Patient is often pale, clammy, and nauseated prior to syncope but is not cyanotic.
      2. Lightheaded feeling is relieved by lying down.
      3. Pulse is slow compared with rapid pulse seen with anaphylaxis.
      4. Hypotension is usually more marked in anaphylaxis.
      5. No respiratory symptoms are present.
   B. Hereditary angioedema (see next section)
IV. Treatment
   A. Inject 0.3 ml of epinephrine 1:1,000 subcutaneously.
   B. If patient is in shock, 1 to 2 ml of epinephrine 1:10,000 may be given intravenously.
   C. Diphenhydramine (Dramamine) 50 mg p.o. or i.v. is given in adults.
   D. Administer supplemental oxygen.
   E. Give intravenous fluids.
   F. If bronchospasm occurs, administer aminophylline intravenously.

G. Corticosteroids may be given, although their effect is not seen immediately.

Hereditary Angioedema

I. Etiology[22]
   A. Most patients have a low level of C1 esterase inhibitor, a component of the complement cascade.
   B. A few patients have normal or high levels of a nonfunctional C1 esterase inhibitor protein.
   C. This results in unchecked cleavage of C4 and C2 by C1 with a consequent low C4 level.
   D. There is a positive family history (dominant inheritance).
II. Signs and symptoms
   A. Produces intermittent angioedema, which is a type of swelling that is larger than urticaria, nonerythematous, and nonpruritic.
   B. Swelling evolves over several hours and lasts 24 to 72 hours, which is longer than the usual acquired or allergic angioedema.
   C. Lesions occur most commonly on the face and extremities.
   D. Laryngeal swelling may lead to airway compromise. In some reports, airway obstruction was responsible for death in 20 to 25% of individuals.
   E. Swelling of the tongue and pharynx can also occur.
   F. Gastrointestinal symptoms of severe cramping, abdominal pain, nausea, and vomiting occur in half the patients and may mimic small bowel obstruction or appendicitis.
   G. Attacks of angioedema usually begin during childhood and increase in frequency during adolescence and early adult life.
   H. Minor trauma precipitates attacks in many patients, although in some cases no initiating event can be determined.
III. Laboratory examination
   A. Serum level of C4 is the screening test.
      1. Abnormally low levels of C4 are found in affected individuals.
      2. Normal or elevated C4 usually rules out this disease.
   B. C1 esterase inhibitor assay is the confirmatory test.
IV. Treatment
   A. Acute attacks[23]
      1. Epinephrine, corticosteroids, and antihistamines have been used separately and together but often do not produce resolution of airway obstruction.
      2. Intubation or tracheotomy may be necessary.
   B. Short-term preventive therapy, e.g., prior to tooth extraction
      1. Administering 2 units of fresh frozen plasma the day before the procedure usually prevents angioedema.

2. Epsilon-aminocaproic acid (EACA) or danazol, an impeded andro-
gen, given 1 to 2 days preoperatively may also be effective.
C. Long-term prophylaxis
1. EACA is indicated for patients with frequent or life-threatening
episodes.
2. Danazol has also proved to be markedly effective.[24]
3. Avoid treating children with the above drugs except in unusual
circumstances.

Bilateral Vocal Cord Paralysis

I. Etiology[25]
A. Recent thyroid or parathyroid surgery
B. Carotid endarterectomy, bilateral
C. Neurologic disorder
D. Malignancy of the thyroid, trachea, or esophagus
E. Jugular foramen syndrome, bilateral
II. Signs and symptoms
A. Depends on etiology
B. Usually inspiratory stridor but remarkably good voice
C. On indirect mirror laryngoscopy or flexible fiberoptic laryngoscopy
the true vocal cords are usually noted to be in the adducted position
and fail to abduct with inspiration.
D. Some people can tolerate bilateral vocal cord paralysis with minimal
symptoms until an upper respiratory infection compromises the airway
a few millimeters more, and then they become extremely dyspneic.
III. Treatment
A. Because most causes of bilateral vocal cord paralysis are not quickly
reversible, most symptomatic patients need a tracheotomy.
B. At a later date, airway widening procedures such as an arytenoidectomy may allow for decannulation of the patient.

Cricoarytenoid Arthritis[26]

I. Etiology
A. Patients usually have florid evidence of rheumatoid arthritis (RA) in
hands and other joints.
B. Approximately 25% of patients with RA have signs and symptoms of
laryngeal involvement, but in only a few of these patients are symptoms
severe.
C. Acute and chronic forms of cricoarytenoid arthritis may be seen.
II. Signs and symptoms
A. Acute cricoarytenoid arthritis

1. Sensation of fullness in throat exacerbated by swallowing or talking
2. Hoarseness
3. Odynophagia
4. Pain in throat with talking or coughing, often radiating to ears
5. Dyspnea
6. Tenderness over thyroid cartilage
7. Erythema over arytenoids
8. Vocal cords normal or slightly edematous but fixed in the adducted position
   B. Chronic cricoarytenoid arthritis
   1. Slight or no hoarseness
   2. Dyspnea
   3. Inspiratory stridor during exacerbation of arthritic process, physical exertion, upper respiratory infection, sleep, or with sedation
   4. Laryngeal examination shows thickening of mucosa over the arytenoids and a narrow airway with inability to abduct vocal cords with inspiration.
   5. Direct laryngoscopy with palpation of the arytenoid cartilage would show fixation to the cricoid cartilage.

III. Treatment
   A. Aspirin or other anti-inflammatory agents
   B. Corticosteroids
   C. Voice rest
   D. Tracheotomy if stridor is prominent and airway is marginal
   E. If tracheotomy is necessary, arytenoidectomy may be considered at a later date as a means to improve the size of the glottic airway so that the patient might be decannulated.

TECHNIQUES FOR MANAGING UPPER AIRWAY OBSTRUCTION

ASSESSMENT OF THE SITUATION

I. In most instances partial rather than total obstruction is present.
   A. Rapidly try to determine the cause by questioning the patient, family, or friends and by performing a cursory physical examination.
   B. Be careful not to turn partial airway obstruction into total obstruction; e.g., turning a child with a tracheal foreign body upside down may cause the object to lodge in the subglottic larynx and result in complete obstruction.
   C. Try the techniques listed in the following sections to improve the airway.

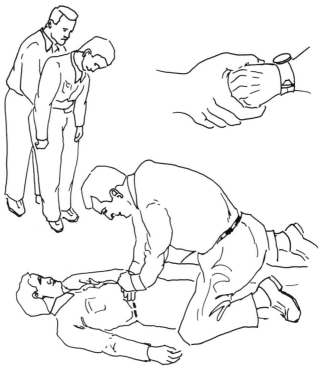

Fig. 8-6. Heimlich maneuver. Approach the standing patient from behind and apply sudden pressure in the epigastrium with clenched fists. Alternatively, kneel beside the supine patient and apply epigastric pressure with the palms of the hands.

II. Total obstruction
    A. If a foreign body is suspected, try the Heimlich maneuver[27] (Fig. 8-6).
    B. If the Heimlich maneuver is unsuccessful, proceed to cricothyroidotomy in the adult or tracheotomy in the young child.
    C. Forced ventilation in the form of mouth-to-mouth or anesthesia mask-to-mouth often provides some ventilation to the lungs while the cricothyroidotomy or tracheotomy is being performed.

III. Respiration has ceased but upper airway obstruction *not* suspected, e.g., cardiopulmonary arrest secondary to a myocardial infarction
    A. Perform the positioning maneuvers (see below) and mouth-to-mouth or mask-to-mouth respiration to rapidly ventilate the patient's lungs.
    B. Make sure that effective cardiac output is being maintained by palpating carotid pulses.
    C. Do not attempt intubation until equipment has been assembled: an endotracheal tube preferably with a stylet, a laryngoscope, and suction.

D. Intubate the patient only after he has been well oxygenated for several minutes.

POSITIONING MANEUVERS

I. The following maneuvers are useful mainly in the unconscious patient who presents with partial upper airway obstruction due to flaccidity of the tongue and pharyngeal muscles.
   A. If the patient exhibits partial airway obstruction in the supine position and if no evidence of a cervical spine injury exists, turn him on his side and place the head sideways and down without a pillow (Fig. 8-4). This head-down position allows the tongue to fall away from the posterior pharyngeal wall and secretions to drain by gravity from the mouth.
   B. If the patient cannot be placed in the lateral or prone position, two other maneuvers are helpful to counteract oropharyngeal obstruction.
      1. The head tilt maneuver (Fig. 8-7) is performed by lifting up the back of the neck while gently pressing the top of the head back and toward the shoulders. *Avoid this maneuver in a patient with a possible cervical spine injury*. This is the position in which mouth-to-mouth respiration is performed.
      2. The jaw thrust maneuver (Fig. 8-5) is performed by placing the fingertips of each hand behind and beneath the angles of the mandible and lifting the mandible forward. This is the position that is used for mask-to-mouth ventilation. The mask is held tightly in position over the nose and mouth with the thumbs.
II. Certain maneuvers are useful mainly in the conscious patient who presents with severe upper airway obstruction from the base of tongue or larynx.
   A. Allow the patient to sit up. This improves pulmonary function and decreases upper airway edema.

Fig. 8-7. Head tilt maneuver. Lift up from the back of the neck while pressing down on the forehead. Avoid this maneuver in a patient with a possible cervical spine injury.

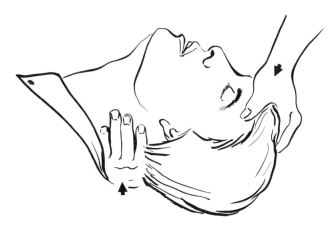

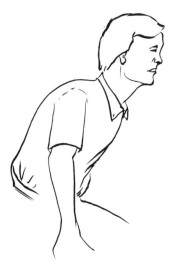

Fig. 8-8. Sitting up and leaning forward with the chin forward opens the upper airway to its maximal extent and also provides good pulmonary ventilation.

B. Encourage the patient to lean forward from the hips and then extend the head from the upper neck so that the chin comes up and forward (Fig. 8-8). This is the position in which children with acute epiglottitis classically present.

AIRWAY STENTS

I. Oral airway (Fig. 8-9)
   A. A curved, hard plastic device inserted between the palate and the tongue

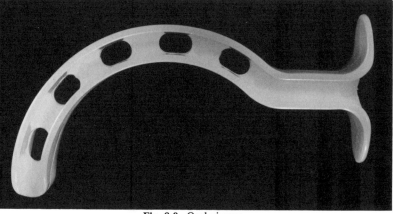

Fig. 8-9. Oral airway.

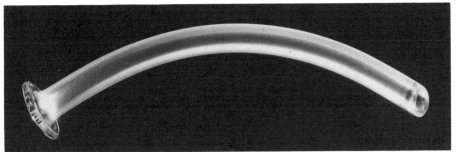

Fig. 8-10. Nasopharyngeal airway.

    B. Used primarily in the unconscious patient to help hold the tongue forward

    C. Also used in the semiconscious intubated patient to prevent him from occluding the tube by biting it

II. Nasopharyngeal airway (Fig. 8-10)

    A. A soft tube placed from the anterior nose to the hypopharynx

    B. Used in the semiconscious and awake patient to allow nasal respiration and to provide ventilation through the region of the oropharynx

OXYGENATION AND VENTILATION

  I. Provide supplemental oxygen while steps are being taken to carry out definitive treatment.

    A. Monitor arterial blood gases to avoid hypercarbia.

    B. Ventilatory assistance may be necessary using manual resuscitation or a mechanical respirator.

 II. Helium–oxygen combination (Heliox) may be a helpful temporary adjunct until definitive treatment can be performed. Helium has lower viscosity than nitrogen and results in less turbulence and improved airflow across the narrowed airway.

ENDOTRACHEAL INTUBATION

   I. Use anesthesia face mask-to-mouth or mouth-to-mouth ventilation until equipment is available.

  II. Equipment includes several sizes of cuffed endotracheal tubes, a stylet, a laryngoscope, and a suction apparatus with both a rigid and flexible suction catheter.

 III. Position patient so that the lower chin and head are slightly extended, i.e., "sniffing" position.

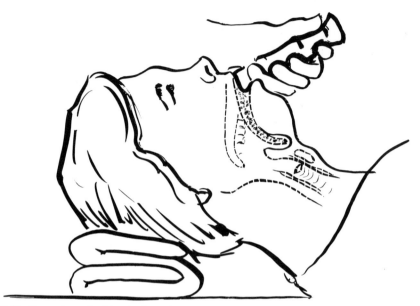

Fig. 8-11. For endotracheal intubation raise the patient's head to straighten the upper airway. The curved laryngoscope blade is placed in the vallecula, thereby elevating the epiglottis and providing direct visualization of the vocal cords.

IV. Insert the laryngoscope with the left hand into the right side of the mouth so that the tongue is to the left of the laryngoscope blade.

V. If a laryngoscope with a curved blade is used, slide it around the base of the tongue into the vallecula and lift it up and away from the operator (Fig. 8-11). This maneuver should lift the epiglottis up and out of the way and the vocal cords should be visible.

VI. If a laryngoscope with a straight blade is used, insert the blade under the epiglottis and lift up.

VII. With the right hand insert the endotracheal tube with stylet into the mouth and through the vocal cords. As the tube is passing the cords, remove the stylet.

VIII. Suction is often needed to clear secretions from the oropharynx and larynx.

IX. If difficulty arises during intubation, do not persist. Ventilate the patient with a mask until oxygenation improves before attempting intubation again.

TRACHEOTOMY

A tracheotomy performed in an uncontrolled situation can be very difficult. If possible, the patient is intubated and the tracheotomy performed over an endotracheal tube.

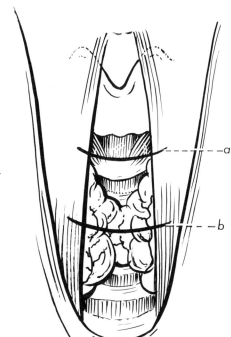

Fig. 8-12. Location of skin incisions for (a) cricothyroidotomy and (b) tracheotomy.

I. Procedure
   A. Calm the patient. Continually explain to the patient what he is going to feel and why. This may alleviate anxiety and helps the procedure go more smoothly.
   B. Supply oxygen as necessary.
   C. If he is able to lie down, have him do so. If not, perform the procedure in the semisitting position.
   D. Place a shoulder roll of rolled sheets or towels under the patient's shoulders in order to extend the neck and bring more of the trachea from the mediastinum into the neck.
   E. Anesthetize the neck midway between the cricoid cartilage and the suprasternal notch using 1% lidocaine with 1:100,000 epinephrine.
   F. With a cautery or scalpel make a transverse incision through the site of injection (Fig. 8-12). In a dire emergency a vertical incision is safer because of less chance for cutting the anterior jugular veins.
   G. After the skin and subcutaneous tissues are divided in transverse planes (avoid cutting the anterior jugular veins), the strap muscles are spread apart with a hemostat in a midline vertical plane and retracted laterally. By staying in the midline and using blunt dissection, vascular structures can be avoided and the tracheotomy can proceed in an orderly fashion.

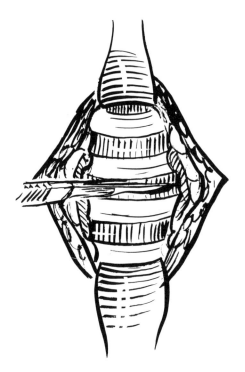

Fig. 8-13. Horizontal incision between the second and third tracheal rings.

H. The isthmus of the thyroid gland may be encountered between the strap muscles and the trachea. The isthmus can be clamped with hemostats, divided, and oversewn. However, it is quicker and safer to retract the isthmus inferiorly or superiorly by placing a hemostat under the isthmus and bluntly dissecting it off of the trachea.

I. Place a tracheal hook below the cricoid or the first tracheal ring and retract superiorly.

J. Make a horizontal incision with a No. 15 scalpel blade between the second and third tracheal rings (Fig. 8-13) and spread the rings apart (Fig. 8-14). Make a vertical tracheal incision in children.

K. In a child with a vertical tracheal incision, one 3-0 silk suture may be placed on each side of the trachea to help locate the tracheal opening in case of accidental dislodgement of the tracheostomy tube during the immediate postoperative period. The "stay" sutures are removed in 3 to 4 days during the first scheduled tracheostomy tube change.

L. A tracheostomy tube whose cuff has been checked for air leaks can then be inserted (Fig. 8-15).

M. Slightly inflate the tracheostomy cuff and secure the tube with a tracheostomy tape that is tied in a square knot. Tracheostomy tapes should not be tied in a bow because they may inadvertently become untied. Sutures that are placed through the skin and the side vents of the trach-

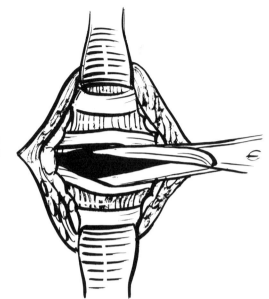

Fig. 8-14. A tracheal spreader is used to separate the rings in order to enlarge the opening.

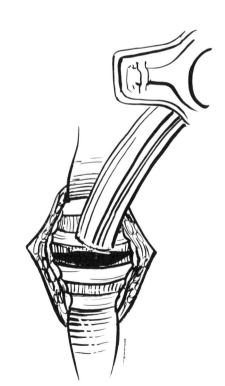

Fig. 8-15. Insertion of a tracheostomy tube.

eostomy tube flange can be used in adults as an alternative to the "stay" sutures described above.

II. Complications

   A. Accidental decannulation is the most common complication of a tracheotomy. It is to avoid this that the tracheostomy tube is stabilized with sutures and/or ties.

   B. Pneumothorax. This is much more common in infants because the pleural apices rise into the neck. After a tracheotomy, a chest x-ray film is immediately obtained to rule out a pneumothorax.

   C. Bleeding. Immediate bleeding is usually the result of injury to the anterior jugular veins. These are ligated with a 3-0 silk suture if accidentally or intentionally severed. Other small bleeding points can be controlled with cautery. Delayed bleeding is usually due to erosion of a great vessel, most seriously the innominate artery. This usually presents as a massive hemorrhage into and around the trachea. It may occur when the tracheotomy is placed too low, usually between the fourth and fifth tracheal rings, and the distal end of the tracheostomy tube erodes into the tracheal wall, or when a necrotizing tracheitis ensues.

   D. Tracheitis sicca. Because the upper airway is now bypassed and cannot perform its role of humidification, the lower trachea becomes very dry. It is important to provide moisture with a tracheostomy collar, a bedside humidifier, or saline instillation. If the humidification is not provided, bleeding and crusting will follow.

   E. Mucous plugs result from inadequate humidification of the tracheal lumen and can be life-threatening if they are not readily recognized. These plugs can be removed with forceps or suctioning and may be accompanied by a small amount of bleeding that is usually not worrisome.

   F. Aerophagia. In the infant, aerophagia may result in gastric distention and vomiting. Nasogastric tube decompression is the treatment of choice.

   G. Hypoxia and death. In an elderly person with chronic airway obstruction, the respiratory center is driven by the patient's hypercarbia. By suddenly reversing this obstruction and providing adequate oxygenation, the CO_2 drive to the respiratory center is eliminated. Apnea and cardiac arrest have been reported.

CRICOTHYROIDOTOMY

Cricothyroidotomy is an alternative to tracheotomy that is used by some because it is easier and quicker to perform, especially for the inexperienced surgeon. The cricothyroid membrane is very superficial and lies just beneath the strap muscles. It is easy to palpate and identify. Cricothyroidotomy is

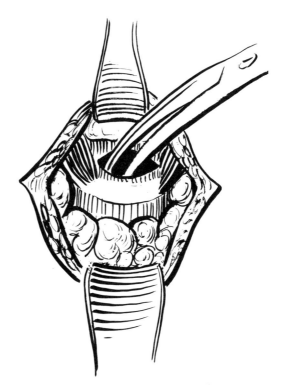

Fig. 8-16. Incision of the cricothyroid membrane.

recommended when a dire emergency exists and there are few, if any, instruments available.

I. Procedure
  A. Extend the neck. Palpate the cricoid cartilage and the lower edge of the thyroid cartilage.
  B. Anesthetize the skin between these two structures and make a horizontal skin incision (Fig. 8-12).
  C. Dissect in the midline and proceed quickly through the cricothyroid membrane (Fig. 8-16).
  D. The airway is entered in the subglottic region, and a tracheotomy tube is inserted.

II. Complications
  The major complication seen with cricothyroidotomy is subglottic stenosis. Because of this concern, a tracheotomy is considered as soon as the patient's condition permits unless it appears that the patient can be decannulated within 48 hours. Subglottic stenosis seems to occur more commonly in children than in adults. The incidence of subglottic stenosis after a cricothyroidotomy is very low if it is changed to a tracheostomy within 48 hours.

REFERENCES

1. Kushner DC, Harris GBC: Obstructing lesions of the larynx and trachea in infants and children. Radiol Clin North Am 16:181, 1978
2. McGovern F: Bilateral choanal atresia in the newborn—a new method of medical management. Laryngoscope 71:480, 1961
3. Maniglia AJ, Goodwin WJ: Congenital choanal atresia. Otolaryngol Clin North Am 14:167, 1981
4. Karma P, Rasanen O, Jarja J: Nasal gliomas: a review and report of two cases. Laryngoscope 87:1169, 1977
5. Ward PH, Thompson R, Calcaterra T, et al: Juvenile angiofibroma: a more rational therapeutic approach based on clinical and experimental evidence. Laryngoscope 84:2181, 1974
6. Weseman CM: Congenital micrognathia. Arch Otolaryngol 69:31, 1959
7. Bluestone CD, Stool SE: Pediatric Otolaryngology. WB Saunders, Philadelphia, 1983
8. Holinger LD: Etiology of stridor in the neonate, infant, and child. Ann Otol Rhinol Laryngol 89:397, 1980
9. Baxter JD: Acute epiglottitis in children. Laryngoscope 77:1358, 1967
10. Committee on Infectious Diseases of the American Academy of Pediatrics: Current status of ampicillin-resistant Hemophilus influenzae type B. Pediatrics 57:417, 1976
11. Cotton RT, Seid AB: Management of the extubation problem in the premature child. Ann Otol Rhinol Laryngol 89:508, 1980
12. Cotton RT: Pediatric laryngotracheal stenosis. J Pediatr Surg 19:699, 1984
13. Leipzig B, Oski FA, Cummings CW, et al: A prospective randomized study to determine the efficacy of steroids in treatment. J Pediatr 94:194, 1979
14. Jones R, Santos JI, Overall JC: Bacterial tracheitis. JAMA 242:721, 1979
15. Petersdorf RG, Adams RD, Braunwald E, et al (eds): Harrison's Principles of Internal Medicine. 10th Ed. p. 1170. McGraw-Hill, New York, 1983
16. Petersdorf RG, Adams RD, Braunwald E, et al (eds): Harrison's Principles of Internal Medicine. 10th Ed. p. 992. McGraw-Hill, New York, 1983
17. Ossoff RH, Wolf AP, Ballenger JJ: Acute epiglottitis in adults: experience with fifteen cases. Laryngoscope 90:1155, 1980
18. Morganstein KM, Abramson AL: Acute epiglottitis in adults. Laryngoscope 81:1066, 1971
19. Hawkins DB, Miller AH, Sachs GB, Benz RT: Acute epiglottitis in adults. Laryngoscope 83:1211, 1973
20. Petersdorf RG, Adams Rd, Braunwald E, et al (eds): Harrison's Principles of Internal Medicine. 10th Ed. p. 855. Mc-Graw Hill, New York, 1983
21. Orange RP, Donsky GJ: Anaphylaxis. In Middleton E, Jr, Reed CE, Ellis EF (eds): Allergy, Principles and Practice. Vol. 2. Mosby, St. Louis, 1978
22. Schneider SB, Atkinson JP: Urticaria and angioedema. In Fitzpatrick TB, Eisen AZ, Wolff K, et al (eds): Update: Dermatology in General Medicine. McGraw-Hill, New York, 1983
23. Frank MM: Hereditary angioedema: the clinical syndrome and its management. Ann Intern Med 84:580, 1976
24. Hosea SW, Santaella ML, Brown EJ, et al: Long-term therapy of hereditary angioedema with danazol. Ann Intern Med 93:801, 1980

25. Tucker HM: Vocal cord paralysis—1979: Etiology and management. Laryngoscope 90:585, 1980
26. Montgomery WW: Cricoarytenoid arthritis. Laryngoscope 73:801, 1963
27. Heimlich HJ, Hoffman KA, Canestri FR: Food choking and drowning deaths prevented by external subdiaphragmatic compression. Ann Thorac Surg 20:188, 1975

9

Nosebleeds

Bruce Leipzig
James Y. Suen ⎯⎯⎯⎯⎯⎯⎯⎯⎯⎯⎯⎯⎯⎯⎯⎯

The etiology of epistaxis may be assigned to any of several categories. These include trauma, hypertension, bleeding disorders, infections, neoplasms, and various miscellaneous disorders.

ETIOLOGY

Trauma

Trauma is the most common cause of epistaxis. Blows to the nose may cause, in addition to fractures, a tear in the nasal mucosa. Digital trauma (nose picking) is a frequent cause of epistaxis especially in children.

Hypertension

Epistaxis is frequently associated with hypertension, especially in older adults who present with severe posterior nasal hemorrhage. The arteriosclerotic vessels lying under a delicate mucosa that is susceptible to drying and cracking often do not retract and clot easily, especially if blood pressure is elevated. Furthermore, the anxiety associated with epistaxis frequently exacerbates the hypertension, and after the acute hemorrhage is controlled the blood pressure may lower spontaneously to some extent. If the diastolic blood pressure is markedly elevated, specific antihypertensive management is indicated, but caution is exercised so as not to reduce the blood pressure excessively, especially if the patient's blood volume is depleted, because hypotension may result in cerebral or cardiac infarction. It is also important not to oversedate the patient because sedation in combination with nasal packing may result in hypoxemia and hypercarbia, especially in the patient with underlying cardiopulmonary pathology.

Although epistaxis is frequently associated with hypertension, the hypertension may not have been the main cause of the epistaxis, especially in the person who was normotensive or only mildly hypertensive prior to the epistaxis. The fear and anxiety of the hemorrhage and the pain associated with its treatment may markedly elevate a person's blood pressure. Bed rest and a mild analgesic may be the only treatment required for this type of hypertension.

Bleeding Disorders

Although most patients with epistaxis have no other hematologic problems, it may be the initial manifestation or a complication of several bleeding disorders:

- Leukemias in children
- Idiopathic thrombocytopenic purpura
- Von Willebrand's disease
- Thrombocytopenia secondary to chemotherapy

Most causes of epistaxis seen in patients with blood dyscrasias are due to quantitative or qualitative abnormalities of platelets. Deficiencies in clotting factors are less common and are screened with a prothrombin time (PT) and partial thromboplastin time (PTT). The PT measures the extrinsic clotting system, and the PTT measures the intrinsic clotting system, specifically factors VIII, IX, XI, and XII. Special factor assays of all the known clotting factors can be performed when indicated.

Infections

Viral, bacterial, and fungal infections of the upper respiratory tract may increase vascularity and capillary fragility and thereby cause epistaxis. Granulomas must also be considered. The infection is treated following the usual and appropriate measures for control of the epistaxis.

Neoplasms

Tumors of the nasopharynx, sinuses, nasal septum, lateral nasal wall, and nasal vestibule are considered as possible causes of the epistaxis if the etiology is not obvious. Sometimes it is impossible to assess the status of the tumor until the nasal packing has been removed and edema has subsided. *A full nasal and nasopharyngeal examination must be performed following treatment for epistaxis.* This may require a repeat examination a month later in the office and is essential to proper treatment. Sinus x-ray films may also be indicated.

Other Etiologies

I. Rendu-Osler-Weber syndrome[1]
   A. Triad of epistaxis, multiple mucosal and cutaneous telangiectasias, and a positive family history of this disease

B. Autosomal dominant transmission
C. Telangiectasias are common in the nasal mucosa as well as the oral cavity, stomach, colon, and lung. Because they lack a muscular coat, they may form arteriovenous fistulas and bleed massively when traumatized.
D. Initial treatment must be gentle and include the use of vasoconstricting agents.
E. Recurrent bleeding is common. Surgical therapy is usually necessary to reduce the frequency and severity of nosebleeds.
II. Hepatic disease
III. Chronic nephritis
IV. Sudden atmospheric pressure changes

EVALUATION

Pertinent History

Although management of profuse epistaxis must take precedence over evaluation of its cause, there are certain salient facts that must be quickly ascertained.
  I. Obtain history from patient or family while preparing the nasal pack tray and during initial observation and examination.
 II. Ask about excess alcohol intake, chronic pulmonary disease, bleeding tendencies or disorders, hypertension, or atherosclerotic cardiovascular disease. These complicating factors carry increased morbidity and mortality.
III. Other pertinent questions
  A. Trauma?
  B. First episode?
  C. Which side?
     Trauma can cause bilateral nose bleeding, but spontaneous epistaxis rarely ever starts bilaterally. It is important to establish which side of the nose started bleeding initially because an anterior nasal pack may cause the bleeding to drain posteriorly and reflux into the opposite nostril so that patients frequently end up with bilateral nasal packs when the bleeding is actually on only one side. Inserting packing gauze can abrade the nasal mucosa and cause other bleeding sites.
  D. Recurrent nosebleeds in the recent or distant past?
  E. Recent sinus infections, nasal or sinus surgery, etc.?
  F. Drug intake, including aspirin, aspirin products, and anticoagulant therapy?

Physical Examination

I. General examination
   A. If the patient gives a history of profuse bleeding or previous serious illness, e.g., heart attack, has had a cerebrovascular accident (CVA), is elderly, or has hypotension, start an intravenous infusion and consider typing and cross-matching blood.
   B. Monitor vital signs frequently.
II. Nasal examination
   A. Place the patient in a sitting position with back and head support.
   B. Use a good light source.
   C. Open the nasal pack tray.
   D. Make sure a good suction apparatus is available.
   E. Have the patient hold an emesis basis to catch the blood (note whether blood is clotted).
   F. Using a nasal suction tip, attempt to remove all blood, examine the nasal cavities carefully, and try to locate the source of bleeding.
   G. If the bleeding has stopped, have the patient blow his nose while in the examining chair to restart the bleeding.

Laboratory Testing

I. Initial tests include a complete blood count (CBC) in order to evaluate the level of anemia and blood loss as well as PT, PTT, bleeding time, and platelet count to screen for bleeding disorders.
II. After a posterior pack is placed, the patient's arterial blood gas levels are obtained.
III. When indicated from the history and physical examination, liver function and renal studies are done.
IV. In children with major or recurrent epistaxis and no history of trauma or surgery to explain it, the diagnosis of von Willebrand's disease must be considered; a low factor VIII level and a prolonged bleeding time are suggestive of this disease, but the response of platelet aggregation to ristocetin is the definitive test.

TREATMENT

Telephone Advice

I. Pinch the nose closed bilaterally with firm pressure by the thumb and forefinger for 10 minutes. This procedure stops most anterior nosebleeds.
II. Sit up with head and neck slightly forward. Many people lie flat on their backs during a nosebleed, which causes the blood to drain into the pharynx and results in spitting up blood or swallowing it and vomiting. This creates more anxiety, increasing the blood pressure and the bleeding.

III. Do not waste time with icepacks or damp cloths on the forehead or back of the neck, as they do little to control nasal bleeding.
IV. If the nosebleed is controlled by the above measures, no further emergency treatment is necessary, but arrangements are made for an intranasal examination.
V. If the nosebleed is uncontrolled during pinching or upon release of the pressure, the patient is told to come to the emergency room immediately.

Emergency Approach to the Bleeding Patient

See Fig. 9-1.
I. All necessary equipment (Table 9-1) is assembled prior to attempting control of hemorrhage.
II. Physician and assistants wear gowns and the patient is draped during the procedure.

Anterior Hemorrhage

I. Mild septal hemorrhage
   A. An anterior bleed is usually found in Little's area (Kiesselbach's plexus), a vascular network near the anterior margin of the nasal septum (Fig. 9-2A). The vascularity of the lateral wall is illustrated in Figure 9-2B.
   B. Treatment
      1. Apply a vasoconstrictor and topical anesthetic to a cotton pledget and place the pledget against the bleeding site for approximately 4 to 5 minutes. This often stops the bleeding or slows it to a trickle.
      2. Silver nitrate can be applied to the bleeding site. The cotton pledget or cotton-tipped applicator is then placed firmly against this area to allow the chemical to work without the blood washing away the silver nitrate (Fig. 9-3). Occasionally, it is necessary to use suction to keep the area clear of blood or to delineate further the need for chemical cautery. Silver nitrate should not be used indiscriminately.
      3. Electrocautery of the mucosa may be performed as an alternative to silver nitrate. Avoid deep contact with the septum, which could result in septal perforation.
      4. Repeated application of cautery to adjacent areas may be required to control an anterior nasal hemorrhage. This is usually due to submucosal excursions of small arterioles with anastomotic connections in Little's area.
      5. Instruct the patient to keep the area moist with antibiotic ointment until it is fully healed as well as to avoid touching the area and avoid blowing the nose.

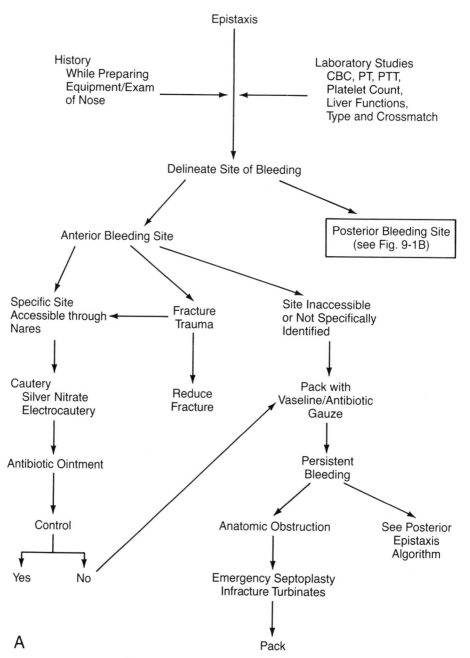

Fig. 9-1. (**A**) Management of nasal bleeding.

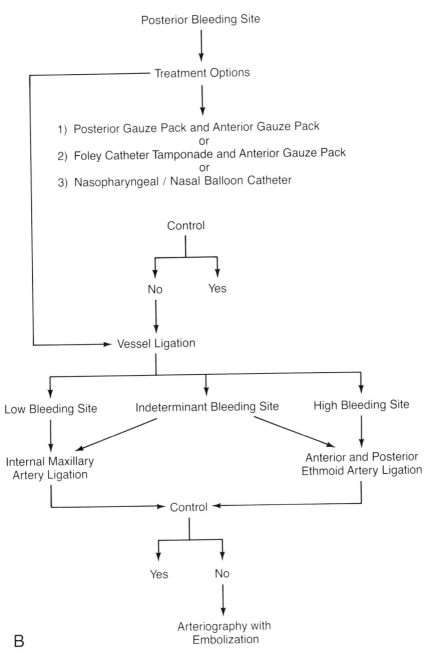

Fig. 9-1. (B) Management of the posterior bleeding site.

TABLE 9-1. ITEMS FOR NASAL PACKING

Equipment	Instruments	Disposable Supplies	Medications
Head mirror and light source (or headlight) Suction machine with nasal aspirators (Frazier suction tip) Emesis basin Electrocautery	Bayonet forceps Nasal speculum Foley catheter Nasostat Hemostats, 3 Syringe	Cotton-tipped applicators Gauze squares, 4 × 4 in. Gauze packing, 0.5 in. Petroleum jelly-saturated nasal packing, 0.5 in. Oxycel pledgets Silk sutures, 2-0 or heavier, or narrow umbilical tape Urethral catheters, 10 French Dental gauze bolster roll Salt pork (for known hematologic disorders)	Silver nitrate sticks 1% Phenylephrine 4% Cocaine (or 2% topical tetracaine) 1% Xylocaine with 1:100,000 epinephrine

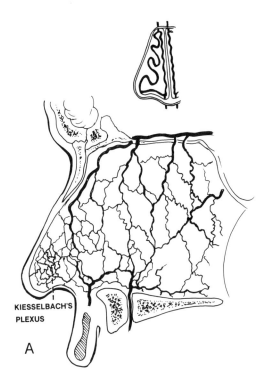

KIESSELBACH'S
PLEXUS

A

Fig. 9-2. (A) Kiesselbach's plexus on
nasal septum. The most common site of
anterior nosebleeds. **(B)** Lateral wall of
nose. Blood supply.

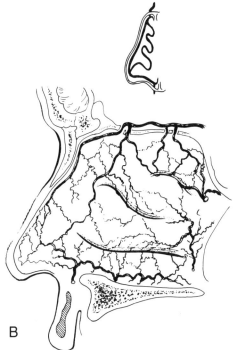

B

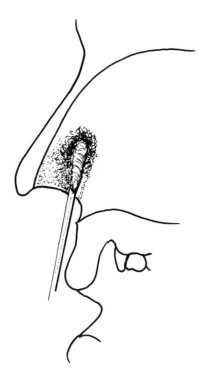

Fig. 9-3. Silver nitrate cautery. A silver nitrate stick is applied directly to the site of bleeding. A cotton-tipped applicator (shown) is then firmly applied to the site.

II. Major anterior nasal hemorrhage

    A. When specific cautery cannot be accurately applied, Oxycel pledgets are packed when the site of bleeding is identified under the inferior or, less commonly, the middle turbinate. Packing the Oxycel from the floor of the nose tightly under the turbinate holds it in place and controls the epistaxis, obviating the need for total anterior gauze packing and/or reinforcement (Fig. 9-4).

    B. If a specific bleeding site cannot be identified, the nose is packed firmly on the side of bleeding with petroleum jelly-soaked gauze. Alternatively, 0.5 inch plain packing, covered with antibiotic ointment, may be used.

        1. Anesthesia

            a) A cotton pledget soaked with an anesthetic and vasoconstrictor solution can be placed inside the bleeding nostril to try to control bleeding while anesthetizing and shrinking the nasal mucosa surfaces.

            b) The topical anesthetic of choice is cocaine, which is both an anesthetic and a vasoconstrictor. No more than 300 mg of cocaine is recommended. An alternative is 1% phenylephrine (Neo-Synephrine) and 2% tetracaine (Pontocaine).

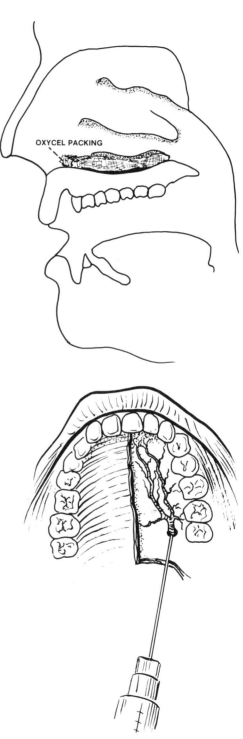

Fig. 9-4. Oxycel packing. The pack is placed under the inferior turbinate, along the floor of the nose. This method may obviate the need for total anterior gauze packing of the nose.

Fig. 9-5. Greater palatine canal injection.

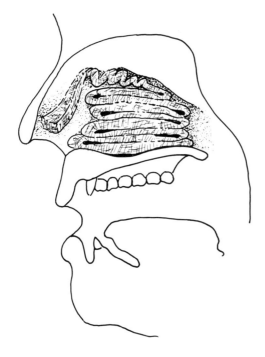

Fig. 9-6. Anterior packing. Packing is placed in a layered fashion beginning inferiorly. Layering prevents dangling of the pack into the nasopharynx and oropharynx and applies gentle, uniform pressure.

c) An alternative treatment involves injecting a solution of 1% lidocaine with 1:100,000 epinephrine into the greater palatine canal through its foramen near the posterior edge of the hard palate. A 25 gauge needle is used to deposit 1 to 2 cc of fluid approximately 2 cm into the canal (Fig. 9-5).

d) Sedation is occasionally necessary for the anxious patient.

2. The pack is placed in horizontal layers beginning along the floor of the nose (Fig. 9-6).

3. Antibiotics, preferably penicillin, are recommended to prevent sinusitis.

C. The pack is removed in approximately 72 hours.

1. On removing the pack, blood may persistently ooze from irritation and an inflammatory response of the nasal mucosa where the pack lay. It often stops without any further treatment. If not, gentle application of a thin layer of Oxycel pledgets often controls this oozing. Patience is required.

2. If significant bleeding occurs during removal of the pack, the packing is reinserted immediately, and either it is left in place for another 3 days or arterial ligation is considered.

3. Humidification and the avoidance of further trauma from nose blowing, picking, or scratching are mandatory for a week after removal of the packing. Irritating blood streaks and nasal mucous secretions may be worrisome but do not require further treatment.

4. Heavy work, sports, and other forms of exertion are avoided for 2 weeks.

Posterior Hemorrhage

I. *It is of critical importance to attempt to identify the area of initial bleeding before packing the nose with a posterior pack.* Many patients initially treated with posterior packing techniques could have been controlled with anterior packing or cautery techniques. Furthermore, should the patient require arterial ligation, identification of the site of bleeding is essential to know which artery or arteries to ligate.
II. Anterior and posterior packs, or a Foley catheter and an anterior pack, control most posterior epistaxis.
III. A Nasostat balloon is effective in some cases. Alternatively, when the patient's medical condition permits, temporary control with balloon catheters is possible followed by immediate arterial ligation as a more comfortable means to control posterior epistaxis.
IV. Foley catheter placement
   A. The catheter is placed transnasally until its tip is barely visible behind the uvula.
   B. Approximately 15 cc of air or a saline solution is injected into the catheter balloon until the balloon feels snug in its position in the nasopharynx.
   C. The catheter is pulled anteriorly, seating the balloon against the posterior choanae (Fig. 9-7). The soft palate will be slightly displaced anteriorly.
   D. An umbilical clamp or hemostat keeps the balloon in its snug position. The clamp is placed over a dental bolster roll to prevent damage to the nasal ala or columella.
V. Technique of posterior packing
   A. Equipment: see Table 9-1.
   B. Anesthesia
      1. The anterior nostril is anesthetized as mentioned in the previous section.
      2. A local anesthetic (2% tetracaine, 10% lidocaine, or any similar anesthetic) is sprayed into the posterior oropharynx to anesthetize it.
   C. Pack placement
      1. The posterior pack is made by rolling a 4 × 4 inch gauze sponge into a 1 inch diameter pack. It is secured with three heavy silk sutures or umbilical cord tapes which are left long.
      2. A 10 French catheter is passed through the nares into the oropharynx and grasped with a hemostat intraorally.

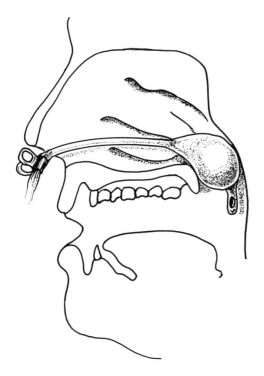

Fig. 9-7. Foley catheter placement. When bleeding is profuse and severe rapid blood loss is of concern, a Foley cathether may be placed in the posterior choana on the side of bleeding as a posterior pack. An anterior pack is then inserted to tamponade the bleeding site.

3. Two of the sutures or tapes are tied to the catheter, and the catheter is pulled back through the nose to deliver the pack through the mouth into the nasopharynx.
4. As the catheter pulls the pack into the nasopharynx, the fingers of the opposite hand can be used to guide the pack until it goes behind the soft palate.
5. The sutures or tapes are pulled until the pack is snugly against the posterior choana (Fig. 9-8A).
6. If both nostrils are being packed, a catheter is passed through each side, and the suture or umbilical tape is pulled through each side of the nose.
7. The third suture or tape should hang visibly in the oropharynx in order to retrieve the pack when it is to be removed.
   D. Completing the packing
      1. After placement of the posterior pack, a unilateral anterior gauze pack is placed according to the technique described earlier (Fig. 9-8B).
      2. To secure the posterior pack the sutures or tapes are then tied over a dental bolster roll in the nasal vestibule (if anterior packing is unilateral) or over the columella (if bilateral anterior packs are present).

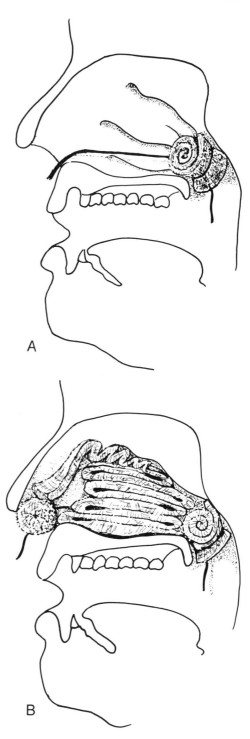

Fig. 9-8. (**A**) Posterior pack. The prepared gauze roll is placed snugly against the choana by pulling the two sutures through the nose. (**B**) An anterior pack is then inserted to tamponade the bleeding site.

E. All patients with both sides of the nose obstructed require low flow oxygen therapy to combat hypoxemia, and antibiotics to prevent sinusitis.[2-4]

F. Repeated observation while the packing is in place is mandatory. Bleeding should be stopped for at least 48 hours and preferably 72 hours prior to pack removal.

Arterial Ligation

I. Indications
   A. Epistaxis uncontrolled by packing
   B. Desire to avoid potential complications of nasal packing (see below) although arterial ligation has its own associated complications
   C. Severe pulmonary disease that would be exacerbated by the hypoxemia and hypercarbia induced by nasal packing

II. Blood supply
   A. Anterior and posterior ethmoid arteries from the ophthalmic division of the internal carotid artery (Fig. 9-2).
   B. Sphenopalatine artery from the internal maxillary division of the external carotid artery (Fig. 9-2).

III. Highlights of technique[5]
   A. The internal maxillary artery is in the pterygomaxillary space behind the maxillary sinus. Create a bony window through the maxillary sinus and expose the pterygopalatine fossa. Use the operating microscope to ligate all of the branches of the internal maxillary artery found in the fossa. Remove nasal packing at the time of arterial ligation and inspect the nose for further bleeding. If bleeding continues, the ipsilateral ethmoid arteries are also ligated.
   B. High lateral wall or high septal bleeding usually is indicative of ethmoid artery hemorrhage. Anterior and posterior ethmoid artery ligation can be performed through a medial canthal incision. The posterior ethmoid artery lies 1 cm posterior to the anterior ethmoid artery and only 4 to 7 mm from the optic nerve. Nevertheless, with careful inspection and identification, this artery can be safely ligated for effective control of epistaxis.
   C. The external carotid artery is the easiest to ligate, but its ligation is *least* successful because of its distal relation to the actual bleeding vessels.
   D. When neither packing nor surgical ligation controls epistaxis, angiography with Gelfoam embolization of the offending artery has been used with some success. This technique is reserved for problem cases of hemorrhage that recur despite exhaustive medical and surgical management.

Patients with Bleeding Disorders

A patient with a bleeding diathesis poses a difficult management problem. The approach to treatment planning is quite different because gauze packs and cauterization may result in a more generalized oozing around the site of treatment. Various agents, including topical Gelfoam packs and Surgicel, which may or may not be soaked in topical thrombin, have been used. There has been some success with the use of bacon fat (or salt pork), which should be kept on hand in the refrigerator in every emergency room and hematology floor of the hospital. A 1.0 to 1.5 cm wide piece of bacon fat is placed against the site of bleeding. The fat swells as it absorbs blood and compresses the bleeding site.[6] It also accelerates coagulation by acting as a platelet substitute. In several days the fat can be easily removed. On occasion, packing may be required and should be both minimal and as gentle as possible. Absorbable Surgicel packing is preferred to gauze.

After control of epistaxis, evaluation of a patient with a bleeding disorder includes the same principles as employed in the diagnosis of any disease process, i.e., history, physical examination, and laboratory testing. Evaluation and replacement of deficient clotting factors may be necessary. Cryoprecipitate or freshfrozen plasma may be necessary in the treatment of hemophilia or von Willebrand's disease.

Hospital Management

I. All patients with bilateral anterior nasal packing and/or posterior packing are hospitalized and given supplemental oxygen. They must be watched closely for hypoxia and possible hypercarbia.

II. Consider admission of all patients who are unstable or at high risk, including those who are elderly, debilitated, or alcoholic with liver disease.

III. Patients who have had repeat packing for control of epistaxis are hospitalized for observation and possible emergency surgical management.

IV. Hypertension, when present, is treated.

V. Basic orders
   A. Bed rest with elevation of head
   B. Humidification of room
   C. Low flow oxygen by face mask for patients with posterior packs
   D. Antibiotics, penicillin preferred
   E. Adequate fluid replacement
   F. Daily hematocrit determination
   G. Ancillary tests based on a more complete history and physical examination
   H. Antihypertensive medications, if indicated

COMPLICATIONS OF TREATMENT

Complications of Nasal Packing

I. Arterial hypoxemia

Patients with anterior and posterior packs in place frequently have hypoxemia. Because patients with epistaxis may often have coexistent cardiovascular and pulmonary disease or borderline liver function, extra care must be taken to avoid hypoxemia. Humidified oxygen at 24 to 40% is recommended by means of a face mask until the packing is removed and palatal edema has subsided. Arterial blood gases are obtained to monitor oxygen therapy. Sedation, when necessary, should be mild.

II. Swallowing difficulty may result from the mass effect of the nasopharyngeal pack.

III. Aspiration of blood or secretions may have occurred during bleeding and packing. Oversedation may also contribute to potential aspiration.

IV. Dislodgement of the pack into the oropharynx and hypopharynx is a known but preventable complication.

V. Eustachian tube obstruction with hemotympanum may result in middle ear effusion and a conductive hearing loss.

VI. Pressure necrosis of the septum and/or turbinate may occur posteriorly as a result of overinflation of balloon-type tamponades or aggressive packing. Similar necrosis may occur from improper techniques of anchoring the posterior packs with sutures or clamps that dig into the mucosa or skin of the nares.

VII. Mucosal tears and new bleeding may occur during the insertion of nasal packs. Careful vasoconstriction and topical shrinking of nasal mucosa prior to placement of the pack allows more adequate visualization and a more gentle technique of nasal packing. In addition, injection of the pterygopalatine canal as described earlier may slow the rate of nasal hemorrhage to allow better visualization. Mucosal tears are often associated with rebleeding upon removal of the pack and may be controlled with cautery or a hemostatic Surgicel gauze pack. These tears are best avoided at the time of initial management.

VIII. Infections

A. Sinusitis due to the obstruction of the sinus ostia is relatively common. Appropriate antibiotic coverage is therefore mandatory until the pack is removed and nasal sinus inflammatory changes resolve.

B. Cavernous sinus thrombosis

C. Orbital cellulitis

IX. Blindness is a rare complication after injection of the pterygopalatine canal.

Complications of Surgery for Vessel Ligation

I. Hypotension and stroke from inadequate fluid replacement prior to or during surgery.
II. Infraorbital nerve anesthesia or paresthesia from surgical trauma during the transantral approach
III. Blindness from inadvertent injury to the optic nerve

REFERENCES

1. McCafferty TV, Kern EB, Lake CF: Management of epistaxis in hereditary hemorrhagic telangiectasia: review of 80 cases. Arch Otolaryngol 103:627, 1977
2. Cassisi NJ, Biller HF, Ogura JH: Changes in arterial oxygen tension and pulmonary mechanics with the use of posterior nasal packing. Laryngoscope 81:261, 1971
3. Lin YT, Orkin LR: Arterial hypoxemia in patients with anterior and posterior nasal packing. Laryngoscope 89:140, 1979
4. Rood SR, Parnes SM, Myers EN, Schramm VL: The Management of Epistaxis. American Academy of Otolaryngology, Rochester, Minn., 1977
5. Chandler JR, Serrins AJ: Transantral ligation of the internal maxillary artery for epistaxis. Laryngoscope 75:1151, 1965
6. Hegwood BB, Davis RB, Yonkers AJ: Treatment of epistaxis with porcine stripped packing. Trans Am Acad Ophthalmol Otolaryngol 82:255, 1976

10

Sudden Sensorineural Hearing Loss

Stephen J. Wetmore ⸺⸺⸺⸺⸺⸺⸺⸺⸺

Sudden unilateral sensorineural hearing loss (SNHL) is often not recognized to be a medical emergency, and the patient is not treated with the urgency that is accorded to someone presenting, for example, with unilateral loss of vision. However, urgent attention is necessary because diseases such as inner ear decompression sickness must be treated within minutes of onset, and other diseases, such as idiopathic sudden hearing loss and oval or round window fistulas, have been shown to have a better prognosis when treated early.

Although sudden SNHL may be due to many etiologies, most investigators believe that viral infections and oval and/or round window fistulas constitute the most common causes. Idiopathic sudden sensorineural hearing loss (ISHL) is most likely due to viral infection. Evidence for this includes the following: The incidence of ISHL does not increase with age as one would suspect if it were due to vascular occlusive disease; steroids have been shown to be effective in the treatment of moderately severe ISHL; histopathologic studies of patients with ISHL show that the changes commonly found are consistent with a viral infection; and the incidence of seroconversions for a number of common viruses in patients with ISHL is higher than in a control population ($p < 0.001$).[1] The second most common cause of sudden SNHL is oval and round window membrane fistula, which is often associated with sudden pressure changes in the ear.

GENERAL INFORMATION

I. Symptoms
    A. The sudden loss of hearing in one ear may be noted upon awakening or may be associated with a popping sensation in the ear followed by roaring tinnitus.
    B. Vertigo may occur.
    C. There is usually no pain.
II. Signs
    A. Nystagmus (if vertigo is present)
    B. Impaired ability to discern spoken words on whisper test (two-syllable words spoken into the patient's ear at varying levels of loudness and the patient asked to repeat the words)

    C. Normal tympanic membrane

    D. No middle ear effusion

III. Tests

    A. Tuning fork tests

       1. Rinne test: Use the 256, 512, and 1,024 Hz tuning forks to compare loudness between the fork placed on the skin over the mastoid cortex and the same fork held in air near the patient's ear canal (Fig. 10-1).

          a) With a conductive hearing loss the patient perceives that the fork placed on the mastoid cortex is louder. With a mild conductive hearing loss the patient states that only the 256 Hz fork seems louder on the mastoid cortex. With a moderate to severe conductive loss all three forks seem louder when held on the bone.

          b) With normal hearing or with a sensorineural hearing loss, the fork held in the air in front of the ear canal sounds louder.

       2. Weber test: The 512 Hz fork is struck and then placed on the patient's forehead or scalp in the midline (Fig. 10-2).

          a) With a unilateral *conductive* hearing loss, the tone is louder in the ear with the conductive hearing loss (worse hearing ear).

          b) With a unilateral *sensorineural* hearing loss, the patient hears the tone louder in the better hearing ear.

    B. Audiogram

       1. Most important test in documenting hearing loss

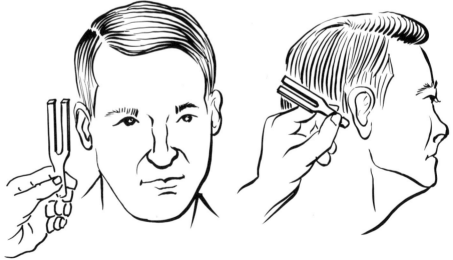

Fig. 10-1. In the Rinne test the patient compares the loudness of the tuning fork transmitted through bone and through air.

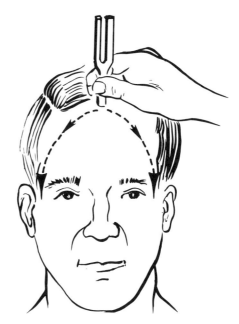

Fig. 10-2. In the Weber test the patient is asked in which ear he hears the tuning fork.

2. Tests the patient's threshold of hearing to pure tones as well as to speech
3. Also tests the patient's ability to understand speech (discrimination score) by asking patient to repeat two-syllable words presented at 40 dB above the threshold of hearing
4. Allows the examiner to determine both the degree of hearing loss and the pattern, e.g., severe high frequency sensorineural loss, moderate low frequency mixed (conductive plus sensorineural) loss
C. Electronystagmography (ENG)
   1. Test of the vestibular system
   2. Performed by attaching electrodes lateral to each eye and looking for nystagmus (Fig. 10-3)

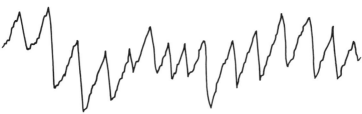

Fig. 10-3. In this tracing of nystagmus the slow component is moving in the upward direction, and the fast component is moving in the downward direction.

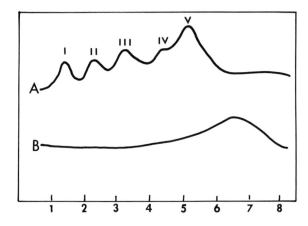

Fig. 10-4. Auditory brainstem response audiometry. (A) A normal response in which all five waves are present and occur within 6 ms of the stimulus. (B) An abnormal response in which wave V is the only discernible wave; it is prolonged to 6.5 ms.

3. Patient is asked to perform several tasks such as following a moving pendulum with his eyes and gazing 20 degrees right and left. He is also placed in various positions, e.g., supine with head left or supine with head hanging over the end of the table, to look for positional nystagmus. Cold and warm water (or air) are then injected into each ear canal to look for a caloric response.
4. Can detect abnormalities of the vestibular portion of the inner ear.
5. May be able to localize the vestibular abnormality either in the brain or in the inner ear.
D. Auditory brainstem response (ABR) audiometry
1. This test is useful in localizing disease occurring in the VIII nerve or brainstem and can be used to detect the threshold of hearing in the higher frequencies.
2. The ear is stimulated by a tone click, and the electrical potentials of the VIII nerve and brainstem that are produced within 10 ms of the stimulus are measured (Fig. 10-4).
3. Because of the low amplitude of these evoked auditory potentials, computer averaging is necessary to distinguish the signal from the background electrical noise.
E. Temporal bone radiographs
1. May be useful for distinguishing ISHL from an acoustic neuroma
2. Look for widening of the internal auditory canal as a sign of a neuroma.
F. Computed tomography (CT scan)
1. A contrast-enhanced CT scan can detect most acoustic neuromas. If the enhanced CT scan is negative for tumor, an air contrast CT scan detects small or intercanalicular tumors.
2. It is usually not necessary in a work-up of ISHL.
G. Serologic test for syphilis

1. FTA-abs remains reactive in inner ear syphilis even if the patient received prior antibiotic therapy.
2. VDRL converts to negative after therapy for systemic syphilis and may therefore be negative in a patient with inner ear syphilis.

DIFFERENTIAL DIAGNOSIS

Idiopathic Sudden Sensorineural Hearing Loss

I. Signs and symptoms
   A. Usually unilateral
   B. Sudden onset: seconds to minutes
   C. Any age group
   D. Often occurs in absence of systemic disease
   E. May be associated with vertigo
   F. Etiology uncertain: viral neuritis vs. mild coagulopathy vs. inner ear membrane break
II. Treatment
   A. A plethora of treatment modalities are espoused.[2] The most promising agents seem to be carbogen[3] and Hypaque,[4] although further studies are needed to prove that these agents are improvements over the spontaneous recovery rate of idiopathic sudden sensorineural hearing loss (ISHL).
   B. Vasodilators
      1. 5% CO_2 (carbogen) dilates intracranial vasculature. A randomized study of carbogen vs. papaverine showed a statistically better hearing gain in the carbogen-treated group 1 year after treatment.[3]
      2. Histamine increases capillary permeability and causes wide swings in blood pressure; it may also be deleterious to the cochlea.
      3. Nicotinic acid has minimal effect on intracranial vessels.
   C. Diatrizoate meglumine (Hypaque). Preliminary results seem promising,[4] but a larger randomized study is needed to determine if intravenous Hypaque therapy achieves better results than the spontaneous recovery rate.
   D. Corticosteroids
      1. A double-blind study[5] showed a 61% recovery rate in a steroid-treated group compared with a 32% recovery rate in a placebo-treated group.
      2. Steroids are most beneficial in patients with a moderate hearing loss.
      3. Almost all patients with mild to moderate midfrequency hearing loss improved in both steroid and placebo groups.
      4. Patients with profound hearing loss received no benefit from steroids.

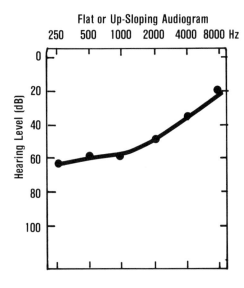

Fig. 10-5. Audiogram associated with a good prognosis for recovery of hearing.

E. Anticoagulants
   1. Low molecular weight dextran and low dose heparin have been given.
   2. They were used on the theory that ISHL is due to thrombosis or capillary sludging.
   3. No good study has shown these drugs to provide any benefit.
III. Prognosis[6]
   A. Factors associated with a *good* prognosis for recovery

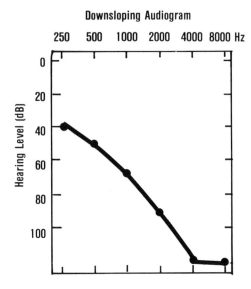

Fig. 10-6. Audiogram associated with a poor prognosis for recovery of hearing.

1. Upwardly sloping audiogram, i.e., hearing worse in low frequencies than in high frequencies (Fig. 10-5)
2. Discrete hearing loss in central portion of audiogram
3. Presence of usable hearing at 8,000 Hz
4. Early diagnosis
   a) Most complete recoveries occur within 14 days of onset.
   b) Some patients take months to improve but often do not obtain a complete recovery.
B. Factors associated with a *poor* prognosis for recovery of hearing
   1. Severe downwardly sloping audiogram (Fig. 10-6)
   2. Severe vertigo
   3. Elevated erythrocyte sedimentation rate
C. The overall recovery rate for hearing in two large series was 45 to 65%.[6,7]

Oval or Round Window Fistula

I. Signs and symptoms
   A. Usually unilateral hearing loss
   B. Sudden onset: seconds to minutes
   C. Any age group
   D. Usually associated with increased inner ear pressure, e.g., heavy lifting, straining, coughing, barotrauma
   E. Vertigo, tinnitus, and headache in the majority of patients[8]
   F. Positive fistula test
      1. Perform by increasing pressure in the external auditory canal with a pneumatic otoscope.
      2. Look for nystagmus beating toward the tested ear or eye deviation to the opposite ear.
      3. Elicits the symptom of vertigo
      4. A fistula may be present even in the face of a negative fistula test.[9]
   G. Presence of positional nystagmus, especially when patient in supine position with involved ear down[9]
   H. ENG usually abnormal
   I. Perilymph fistula at oval or round window noted at surgery
II. Treatment
   A. Medical management
      1. Bed rest, for 5 days
      2. Recommended when patient seen early after onset of symptoms
      3. Head of bed elevated 30 to 40 degrees
      4. Sedation
      5. Stool softeners—no straining

      6. If symptoms clear after 5 days of bed rest, the patient is allowed limited activity for 10 days; thereafter the patient is slowly allowed to resume normal activities.

  B. Surgical management

    1. Indications

      a) Failed medical therapy

      b) Symptoms of more than 1 month's duration

    2. Exploratory tympanotomy under local anesthesia

      a) Fistulas not readily apparent may become more evident by lowering the head of the operating table and asking the patient to perform a Valsalva maneuver.

      b) If a fistula is identified, it is sealed with fascia, fat, or perichondrium.

III. Prognosis

  A. Majority of patients recover from hearing loss and/or vertigo. The efficacy of medical management is not known, and recovery may be spontaneous.

  B. In the group of patients undergoing surgical therapy, approximately half have cessation of vertigo, but most do not recover from the hearing loss.[8,9]

    1. The surgical group usually contains patients with poorer prognosis.

    2. The medical group may contain patients who actually have ISHL rather than a confirmed fistula.

Meniere's Disease

  I. Signs and symptoms

    A. Initial episode of hearing loss, tinnitus, and vertigo may present like ISHL.

    B. Cochlear Meniere's disease, a variant of classic Meniere's disease, presents with fluctuating sensorineural hearing loss.

  II. Treatment and prognosis

    See Chapter 11.

Otosyphilis[10]

  I. Signs and symptoms

    A. Congenital otosyphilis[11]

      1. Onset of hearing loss in children is usually very sudden, bilaterally symmetrical, profound, and unaccompanied by vertigo.

      2. Onset in adults may be abrupt and bilateral but is usually asymmetrical.

  3. In adults the hearing loss often fluctuates and is usually associated with episodic vertigo and tinnitus.
  4. Other signs of congenital syphilis are usually present, e.g., interstitial keratitis, Hutchinson's teeth, and sabre shins.
  5. FTA-abs is positive.
  6. Pathophysiology is osteitis of otic capsule with secondary endolymphatic hydrops.
 B. Acquired otosyphilis[12]
  1. Age usually 40 to 60 years
  2. Often present with unilateral hearing loss but other ear eventually becomes involved
  3. Often present with symptoms compatible with Meniere's disease
  4. FTA-abs is positive
  5. No stigmata of congenital syphilis
II. Treatment
 A. Corticosteroids
  1. Prednisone 80 mg every other day
  2. May require weeks to months of therapy
  3. Slowly taper to lowest possible dose if significant hearing gain is documented on audiometry.
  4. A significant audiologic response is defined as a 15% improvement in the pure tone average or a 15% improvement in the speech discrimination score.
  5. If hearing does not improve after 4 weeks of therapy, the corticosteroids are rapidly tapered and discontinued.
 B. Antibiotics: long-term penicillin therapy, e.g., benzathine penicillin G, 2.4 million units i.m. each week for 3 months
III. Prognosis
 A. Approximately 35% of patients obtain improved hearing with treatment but only one-half of those maintain improvement for 1 year.[13]
 B. Patients with acquired otosyphilis have a 43% initial response rate and a 25% lasting response rate.[14]
 C. Patients with congenital otosyphilis have a 20% initial response rate and no lasting response rate.[14]

Acoustic Neuroma

I. Signs and symptoms
 A. Sudden unilateral hearing loss is an uncommon presentation of an acoustic neuroma but may occur in as many as 17% of cases.[15]
 B. Tinnitis is usually present.
 C. Unsteady sensation rather than whirling vertigo often occurs.

D. Audiometry with acoustic reflex tests, ABR, ENG, and radiographs of internal auditory canals are screening tests. If suspicion is high, an intravenous contrast-enhanced CT scan is the definitive test for a large tumor, and an intrathecal air contrast CT scan is the definitive test for a small tumor.

II. Treatment and prognosis
  A. Surgical excision of tumor
  B. Rarely preserves hearing

Inner Ear Decompression Sickness[16]

I. Signs and symptoms
  A. Seen in deep sea divers who ascend too rapidly
  B. Hearing loss and/or vertigo due to bubbles of gas forming in the inner ear
  C. Possibly other symptoms of decompression disease, e.g., pains in the knees, shoulder, back, or substernal region
II. Treatment and prognosis
  A. Immediately recompress patient to a depth of at least 3 atmospheres (100 feet) deeper than the depth at which symptoms began.
  B. Switch back to helium–oxygen rather than air.
  C. Divers who are recompressed within 40 minutes after onset of symptoms have no residual dysfunction; if treatment is delayed more than 70 minutes, prognosis for recovery of inner ear function is poor.

REFERENCES

1. Wilson WR, Veltri RW, Laird N, Sprinkle PM: Viral and epidemiologic studies of idiopathic hearing loss. Otolaryngol Head Neck Surg 91:653, 1983
2. Mattox DE: Medical management of sudden hearing loss. Otolaryngol Head Neck Surg 88:111, 1980
3. Fisch U: Management of sudden deafness. Otolaryngol Head Neck Surg 91:3, 1983
4. Emmett JR, Shea J: Diatrizoate meglumine (Hypaque) treatment for sudden hearing loss. Laryngoscope 89:1229, 1979
5. Wilson WR, Byl FM, Laird N: The efficacy of steroids in the treatment of idiopathic sudden hearing loss. Arch Otolaryngol 106:772, 1980
6. Mattox DE, Simmons FB: Natural history of sudden sensorineural hearing loss. Ann Otol Rhinol Laryngol 86:463, 1977
7. Byl FM: Sudden hearing loss: eight years experience and suggested prognostic table. Laryngoscope 94:647, 1984
8. Thompson JN, Kohut RI: Perilymph fistulae: variability of symptoms and results of surgery. Otolaryngol Head Neck Surg 87:898, 1979
9. Singleton GT, Karlin MS, Post KN, Bock DG: Perilymph fistulas: diagnostic criteria and therapy. Ann Otol Rhinol Laryngol 87:797, 1978

10. Steckleberg JM, McDonald TJ: Otologic involvement in late syphilis. Laryngoscope 94:753, 1984
11. Karmody CS, Schuknecht HF: Deafness in congenital syphilis. Arch Otolaryngol 83:18, 1966
12. Becker GD: Late syphilitic hearing loss: a diagnostic and therapeutic dilemma. Laryngoscope 89:1273, 1979
13. Zoller M, Wilson WR, Nadol JB: Treatment of syphilitic hearing loss: combined penicillin and steroid therapy in 29 patients. Ann Otol Rhinol Laryngol 88:160, 1979
14. Dobbin JM, Perkins JH: Otosyphilis and hearing loss: response to penicillin and steroid therapy. Laryngoscope 93:1540, 1983
15. Morrison AW: Management of Sensorineural Deafness. p. 180. Butterworth, London, 1975
16. McCormick JG, Holland WB, Brauer RW, Holleman IL Jr: Sudden hearing loss due to diving and its prevention with heparin. Otolaryngol Clin North Am 8:417, 1975

11

Vertigo

Stephen J. Wetmore

Dizziness is a general term that includes the terms vertigo, unsteadiness, and light-headedness. Vertigo is a more limited term and refers to the hallucination of motion or the sensation of spinning. Vertigo can result from either peripheral vestibular conditions (inner ear) or from central nervous system (CNS) problems.

DIAGNOSIS

History

The history is the most important aspect in the diagnosis of vertigo.
I. Dizziness
  A. Type of dizziness
    1. Vertigo
      a) Sensation of motion
      b) Usually seen with inner ear disease
      c) Possibly from CNS disease
    2. Unsteadiness
      a) May occur with inner ear or VIII nerve disease
      b) Can also occur with CNS disease, peripheral neuropathies, anemia, generalized debility and a host of other conditions
    3. Light-headedness
      Can result from a myriad of conditions including inner ear abnormalities
  B. Duration
    1. Inner ear problems tend to be episodic with duration of seconds to days.
    2. CNS problems may be episodic or constant.
  C. Severity
    Inner ear problems tend to cause a more severe effect than do CNS problems.
  D. Precipitating event
    1. Dizziness precipitated by body posture changes, sudden pressure changes, and changes in diet, e.g., increased salt intake, tends to be due to inner ear problems.

2. Dizziness brought on by turning the head may be due to inner ear problems but can also be due to brainstem hypoxia caused by occluding or twisting a major blood vessel in the neck or from cervical vertigo precipitated by stimulating the spinovestibular proprioceptors in the vertebral column.

3. Conversely, if no eliciting event can be discovered, inner ear problems *cannot be ruled out.*

II. Associated symptoms which point *to* an inner ear etiology:
   A. Hearing loss
   B. Otalgia
   C. Otorrhea
   D. "Fullness" in the ear

III. Associated symptoms which point *away* from an inner ear etiology:
   A. Syncope or "black out" spells
   B. Loss of vision
   C. Irregular pulse
   D. Bowel or urinary incontinence
   E. Seizures

IV. Symptoms which may be seen with either inner ear or CNS problems (or both):
   A. Head trauma
   B. Abnormal eye movements (nystagmus)

Physical Examination

   I. Otolaryngologic examination
   II. Ophthalmologic examination—looking for nystagmus
   III. Screening neurologic examination
      A. Cranial nerves
      B. Motor function
      C. Sensory modalities, e.g., touch, pain, temperature
      D. Balance and coordination
         1. Finger to nose test
         2. Rapid alternating movements—hands, feet
         3. Gait
         4. Tandem gait
         5. Romberg test
      E. Reflexes

Tests

   I. Vestibular function
      A. Caloric test
         1. The patient is placed in the supine position but with the head elevated 30 degrees.

2. The ice water caloric test is performed by injecting 5 ml of cold water into the ear canal over a 5 second period.
3. Look for nystagmus beating toward the opposite ear and measure duration (acronym is COWS: cold water, opposite ear—warm water, same ear).
4. If the nystagmus elicited on one side is diminished or absent compared with the contralateral side, the ear with the diminished response is usually the abnormal ear.
5. Ask patient how the elicited vertigo compares in nature and severity with his spontaneous dizziness.
6. This test produces optimal responses if the patient is performing a mentally alerting task such as counting backward from 100 by 7s, i.e., 100 . . . 93 . . . 86 . . . 79 . . .
7. The caloric test is best performed as part of electronystagmography (ENG) so that the slow wave velocity of the nystagmus response can be measured. Slow wave velocity is a more accurate measurement than is duration of nystagmus.

B. Dix-Hallpike test (Fig. 11-1)
1. This is used to diagnose benign paroxysmal positional vertigo.
2. The patient, who is seated on an examination table, is rapidly placed in a supine position with his head hanging beyond the end of the table and facing either right or left.

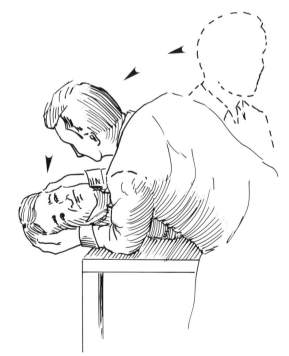

Fig. 11-1. Dix-Hallpike test for benign paroxysmal positional vertigo. The examiner quickly places the patient from a sitting position to a supine position with the patient's head hanging over the edge of the table and turned either to the right or to the left.

3. The examiner looks for nystagmus elicited by this quick position change and asks the patient if he is dizzy.
4. If nystagmus or dizziness occurs, the examiner repeats the test to see if the response diminishes the second time.
5. If no dizziness or nystagmus occurs, the test is repeated with the face turned to the opposite direction.
   C. Electronystagmography
   1. This is a test of the vestibular system that is performed by attaching electrodes lateral to each eye and looking for nystagmus on a strip chart recording (see Fig. 10-2).
   2. The caloric test can be performed by injecting cold and warm water (or air) and measuring the slow wave velocity of the nystagmus.
   3. The Dix-Hallpike test, other positional tests, gaze test, pendulum tracking test, and optokinetic reflex testing can be performed and objectively recorded.
   4. ENG may be able to differentiate CNS from inner ear abnormalities and may be able to pinpoint which ear is causing the problem.
 II. Audiogram
   A. Precise test of auditory function
   B. May be able to differentiate VIII nerve from inner ear abnormalities with special audiometric tests
III. Auditory brainstem response (ABR) audiometry (see Ch. 10)
   A. Accurate test of VIII nerve and brainstem function
   B. Useful for detecting acoustic neuroma and multiple sclerosis
 IV. Blood tests
   A. Complete blood count (CBC): anemia
   B. Thyroid function tests: hypothyroidism, a rare cause of vertigo
   C. Glucose assay: diabetes mellitus and reactive hypoglycemia. May need a 5-hour glucose tolerance test to detect reactive hypoglycemia.
   D. VDRL and FTA-abs: syphilis (see Ch. 10)
  V. X-ray examination
   A. Mastoid films: look for asymmetry in the size of the internal auditory canals: acoustic neuroma
   B. Computed tomography (CT scan): acoustic neuroma

MANAGEMENT OF VERTIGO

Acute Episode of Vertigo, Nausea, and Vomiting

 I. Vestibular suppressants
   A. Intravenous diazepam (Valium) 5 to 10 mg injected slowly over a 3- to 5-minute period produces a reduction in symptoms.
   B. The above dose may have to be repeated in a few hours if severe symptoms recur.

C. Diazepam 5 mg P.O. q8h can be used to treat acute vertigo that is less severe.

D. Prochlorperazine (Compazine) 5 to 10 mg i.m. or 25 mg per rectum is an alternative for severe vertigo.

E. Vagolytic agents such as atropine may also be useful in the acute attack of vertigo.

II. Bed rest in a quiet room

Chronic Vertigo

Diagnose the disease process and treat accordingly.

DIFFERENTIAL DIAGNOSIS

See Table 11-1.

INNER EAR DISORDERS

Vestibular Neuronitis[1]

I. Symptoms

A. Acute onset of vertigo

B. Duration of vertigo 2 to 6 days, but unsteadiness may persist for 6 to 8 weeks

TABLE 11-1. DIFFERENTIAL DIAGNOSIS OF VERTIGO

	Whirling Vertigo	Unsteadi-ness	Hearing Loss	Abnormal ABR	Abnormal ENG
Inner ear disorders					
Vestibular neuronitis	+	−	−	−	+
Meniere's disease	+	−	+	−	+/−
Oval or round window fistula	+	+	+	−	+
Toxic labyrinthitis	+/−	+	+/−	−	+
Serous labyrinthitis	+	+	+	−	+/−
Inner ear concussion	+	+	+	−	+/−
Benign paroxysmal positional vertigo	+	−	−	−	+
Central nervous system disorders					
Acoustic neuroma	−	+	+	+	+
Vertebral basilar artery insufficiency	+	−	−	−	+/−
Multiple sclerosis	+	+	−	+	+

    C. Often associated or preceded by an upper respiratory infection
    D. Vegetative symptoms of nausea and vomiting
    E. Absence of other symptoms
II. Signs
    A. Nausea and vomiting
    B. Spontaneous nystagmus toward the uninvolved ear
    C. Absence of other neurologic signs
III. Tests
    A. Caloric test: abnormal
    B. ENG
        1. Preferable to caloric test
        2. Shows hypoactive or absent caloric response in one ear
        3. May be abnormal months after the vertigo subsides
    C. Audiogram: usually normal
IV. Differential diagnosis
    A. Meniere's disease
        1. Duration of vertigo shorter in Meniere's disease
        2. Other symptoms: tinnitus, hearing loss, ear fullness
        3. Recurrent
    B. Toxic labyrinthitis
        1. Vertigo usually less severe
        2. Usually can identify etiologic factor
V. Treatment
    Vestibular suppressants are used.
    A. Diazepam, initially 5 to 10 mg I.V. push slowly; given by mouth when symptoms begin to subside
    B. Meclizine 25 mg q8h sometimes helpful after severe vertigo abates
VI. Natural course of disease
    A. Initial episode may require bed rest for 2 to 5 days.
    B. It may recur, especially in older individuals.
    C. Motion intolerance may last for months.

Meniere's Disease

I. Symptoms
    A. Vertigo lasting 20 minutes to 24 hours
    B. Tinnitus usually exacerbated during the episode
    C. Fluctuating hearing loss
    D. Full sensation in the ear or head
    E. Motion intolerance between vertiginous episodes
II. Signs
    A. Nausea and vomiting
    B. Nystagmus
    C. Hearing loss

III. Tests
  A. Audiogram
    1. Low frequency sensorineural hearing loss is most common.
    2. Early in the course of the disease the hearing characteristically fluctuates and may return to normal between episodes.
    3. Later in the disease, the hearing may become progressively worse.
  B. ENG: nonspecific abnormalities
  C. FTA-abs: to rule out syphilis, which may present in a fashion identical to Meniere's disease
IV. Differential diagnosis
  A. Inner ear syphilis: positive FTA-abs
  B. Late effect of inner ear trauma: scarring in inner ear may produce symptoms identical to Meniere's disease.
 V. Treatment
  A. Acute attacks
    1. Vestibular suppressants, e.g., diazepam 5 to 10 mg I.V. for severe episodes.
    2. Bed rest
  B. Between acute attacks
    1. Diuretic, e.g., hydrochlorothiazide 50 mg daily
    2. Low salt diet
    3. Vestibular suppressants, e.g., diazepam, 2 to 5 mg q8h
    4. Eighty percent of patients obtain partial or complete relief of symptoms with medical therapy.
  C. Surgical therapy
    1. Endolymphatic sac surgery, performed via a mastoidectomy, has a 60% long-term success rate in alleviating vertigo.[2]
    2. Vestibular nerve section, performed via a middle fossa craniotomy, has a 96% long-term success rate for controlling vertigo.[3]
    3. Labyrinthectomy has a 93% success rate but destroys hearing.[3]
VI. Natural course of disease and pathophysiology
  A. Episodic nature
  B. Cochlear variant: episodic fluctuating hearing loss, tinnitus, and ear fullness but without vertigo
  C. Vestibular variant: episodic vertigo without hearing loss
  D. Bilateral ear involvement in as many as 30% of cases
  E. Endolymphatic hydrops is the pathologic correlate, with ballooning of the cochlear duct.
  F. Course of the disease is variable.
    1. Some patients have episodes of vertigo which occur months to years apart with minimal progression of hearing loss.
    2. Some patients have a 10- to 15-year history of episodes of vertigo which are months apart but which eventually stop recurring; the hearing loss, however, is often progressive.

3. Other patients experience frequent (less than 1 week apart) episodes of vertigo which incapacitate them: Hearing is often moderately impaired.
4. It is not known if early surgical intervention prevents progression of this disease.

Oval or Round Window Fistula

See also Chapter 10.
I. Symptoms
  A. Vertigo
  B. History of pressure change
    1. Sneeze
    2. Strain
    3. Scuba diving
  C. Hearing loss, sensorineural
    1. Incidence varies
    2. Severity varies
II. Signs
  A. Unsteadiness
  B. Nausea and vomiting
  C. Hearing loss
  D. Nystagmus
III. Tests
  A. Fistula test: use the pneumatic otoscope to change pressure in the external auditory canal and look for either nystagmus or eye deviation.
  B. Audiogram
  C. ENG: usually abnormal
IV. Differential diagnosis
  A. Initial episode of Meniere's disease
  B. Vestibular neuronitis
V. Treatment
  A. Bed rest
  B. Vestibular suppressants
  C. Surgical closure of fistula
VI. Course of disease and pathophysiology
  A. Vertigo usually subsides with bed rest or surgical intervention.
  B. Hearing loss, if present, may not improve.[4]
  C. Pathophysiology consists of an oval or round window fistula resulting in altered inner ear fluid dynamics.

Toxic Labyrinthitis (Ototoxic Drug Effect)

I. Symptoms
  A. Gradual onset of vertigo
  B. Unsteadiness

    C. Hearing loss

    D. History of ototoxic drug ingestion especially aminoglycosides

        1. Symptoms may occur during ototoxic drug therapy or may not present until weeks later.

        2. Often patient is asymptomatic while in bed.

  II. Signs

    A. Ataxia

    B. Nystagmus

    C. Hearing loss

        1. The hearing loss is of a high frequency bilateral sensorineural nature.

        2. Some ototoxic agents (e.g., gentamicin) predominantly produce vestibular symptoms whereas others (e.g., neomycin) predominantly produce hearing loss.

 III. Tests

    A. ENG shows bilateral hypoactive caloric responses.

    B. Audiogram may show a high frequency bilateral sensorineural hearing loss that sometimes progresses into the middle frequencies.

 IV. Differential diagnosis

    A. Multiple sclerosis

    B. Brain tumor: look for other neurologic signs

  V. Treatment

    A. Further avoidance of ototoxic drugs

    B. Maximal use of visual and proprioceptive cues

 VI. Course of illness and pathophysiology

    A. CNS compensation may result in improvement of symptoms.

    B. Associated hearing loss, if present, may not improve.

    C. There is a toxic effect on vestibular hair cells of semicircular canals and otolithic membranes.

Serous Labyrinthitis

  I. Symptoms

    A. Vertigo

    B. Unsteadiness

    C. Hearing loss

    D. Preceding or concomitant ear injury

        1. Acute suppurative otitis media

        2. Stapedectomy

  II. Signs

    A. Nystagmus

    B. Ataxia

    C. Hearing loss

    D. Red, bulging tympanic membrane or purulent otorrhea
    E. Recent ear surgery

III. Tests
    A. ENG may show unilateral hypoactivity and spontaneous nystagmus
    B. Audiogram may show a mixed conductive and sensorineural hearing loss

IV. Differential diagnosis
    A. Toxic labyrinthitis
    B. Vestibular neuronitis
    C. Oval or round window fistula
    D. Bullous myringitis
       1. Otalgia
       2. Multiple bullae on tympanic membrane and medial external auditory canal wall
       3. Occasionally, reversible sensorineural hearing loss with vertigo[5]

V. Treatment
    A. Associated with acute suppurative otitis media
       1. Antibiotics
       2. Myringotomy
    B. Associated with recent surgery
       1. Close observation
       2. Vestibular suppressants

VI. Course of illness and pathophysiology
    A. Usually complete resolution
    B. Rarely recurs
    C. Toxic effect of nearby inflammation

Inner Ear Concussion

  I. Symptoms and signs
    A. Recent head injury
    B. Vertigo
    C. Unsteadiness
    D. Hearing loss
    E. Headache
    F. Nystagmus

  II. Tests
    A. ENG may show positional nystagmus or benign paroxysmal positional nystagmus.
    B. Audiogram may show unilateral sensorineural hearing loss, usually in high frequencies.

III. Differential diagnosis
    A. Serous labyrinthitis
    B. Toxic labyrinthitis

C. Cervical vertigo

D. Subdural hematoma

IV. Treatment

  A. Vestibular suppressants

  B. Labyrinthine exercises (see Benign Paroxysmal Positional Vertigo, Treatment, below). Instruct patient to perform tasks which result in vertigo in order to allow central vestibular compensation to occur more rapidly.

V. Course of illness: may last weeks to months

Benign Paroxysmal Positional Vertigo

I. Symptoms and signs

  A. Classic vertigo

    1. Vertigo upon assuming a particular position

    2. Latency period of a few seconds prior to vertigo

    3. Severe vertigo lasting 5 to 30 seconds

    4. Fatigue of response upon repetition, i.e., weaker response

    5. Diseased ear is the one in the "down" position

  B. Nonclassic vertigo

    1. Vertigo upon assuming a particular position

    2. No latency

    3. Nonfatigable

  C. Absence of other symptoms

  D. Sometimes associated with inner ear concussion and whiplash injuries

  E. Nystagmus induced with positioning of patient

II. Tests

  A. Dix-Hallpike test

  B. ENG

III. Differential diagnosis

  A. Orthostatic hypotension

  B. Hyperventilation syndrome

  C. Cervical vertigo, elicited by twisting head or torso rather than by positioning head with one ear down

IV. Treatment

  A. Labyrinthine exercises

    1. Place patient in lateral position to produce vertigo (Fig. 11-2).

    2. Then place patient in sitting position.

    3. Then place patient in position opposite to position 1.

    4. Repeat steps 1 to 3 until symptoms stop.

    5. Repeat steps 1 to 4 four times daily until patient is free of symptoms for 2 to 3 days. This usually requires 3 to 14 days of treatment.[6]

  B. Vestibular suppressants

  C. Vestibular nerve section (singular neurectomy)[7]

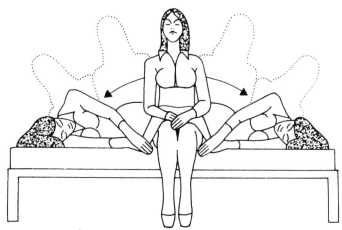

Fig. 11-2. Labyrinthine exercises. (Brandt T, Daroff RB: Physical therapy for benign paroxysmal positional vertigo. Arch Otolaryngol 106:484, 1980.)

      1. For patients whose symptoms are unresponsive to other therapy
      2. Rarely needed
 V. Natural course and pathophysiology
    A. Usually subsides in weeks to months
    B. May become chronic
    C. The pathophysiology is thought to be due to otoconia from the utricular macula falling onto the crista of the posterior semicircular canal and producing excessive stimulation of the posterior semicircular canal whenever that canal is in a certain position.

CNS DISORDERS

Acoustic Neuroma

  I. Symptoms
    A. Unsteadiness rather than whirling vertigo
    B. Unilateral sensorineural hearing loss
    C. Tinnitus
    D. Symptoms of increased intracranial pressure, e.g., headache and vomiting, are unusual and occur late in the course of this disease.
 II. Signs
    A. Unilateral hearing loss
    B. Other neurologic signs such as ataxia, hypoactive corneal reflex, and ipsilateral facial hypesthesia for pain, temperature, and touch occur relatively late in the course of this disease.
III. Tests

A. Audiogram
    1. Most patients exhibit a unilateral hearing loss.
    2. Bilateral hearing loss may be present in the forme fruste of von Recklinghausen's disease.
    3. The speech discrimination score is often lower than would be expected from the pure tone hearing threshold.
    4. The acoustic reflex test and/or the acoustic reflex decay test are usually abnormal.
B. Auditory brainstem response (ABR) audiometry (see Ch. 10)
    1. ABR is abnormal in 90% of patients with acoustic neuromas.[8]
    2. A standard audiogram is necessary to adjust ABR results for the degree of hearing loss.
C. ENG: unilateral hypoactive caloric response in most neuroma patients
D. X-ray examination
    1. Plain films or tomograms of the internal auditory canal often show erosion or widening of the canal.
    2. CT scan is the definitive test.
        a) An intravenous contrast-enhanced CT scan detects most larger neuromas.
        b) If this scan is negative but a neuroma is still suspected, an air contrast CT scan can be obtained. This study detects small (intercanalicular) tumors. Because this study requires a lumbar puncture, it is not requested if elevated intracranial pressure is suspected.
IV. Treatment and prognosis
    A. The tumor is surgically excised.
    B. Only rarely can hearing be preserved in the involved ear.
    C. Although the acoustic neuroma is usually a slow-growing benign tumor, if untreated it eventually results in severe neurologic disability and death.

Vertebral Basilar Insufficiency[9]

I. Symptoms
    A. Vertigo
        1. Episodic
        2. Sometimes precipitated by postural hypotension, Stokes-Adams attacks, or mechanical compression from cervical spondylosis.
    B. Slurred speech
    C. Nausea and vomiting
    D. Visual disturbances
II. Signs
    A. Nystagmus

    B. Subtle signs of residual neurologic dysfunction

    C. Hypertension

    D. Atherosclerosis

    E. Diabetes mellitus

    F. Hyperlipidemia

III. Tests

    A. ENG

    B. Electroencephalography (EEG): abnormal in one-third of patients

IV. Differential diagnosis

    A. Posterior-inferior cerebellar artery infarction (Wallenberg syndrome)

        1. Ipsilateral facial hypesthesia for pain and temperature

        2. Ipsilateral paralysis of palate, pharynx, and larynx

        3. Ipsilateral Horner's syndrome: miosis, ptosis, and decreased sweating

        4. Ataxia

        5. Contralateral body hypesthesia for pain and temperature

    B. Anterior-inferior cerebellar artery infarction

        1. Ipsilateral hearing loss

        2. Ipsilateral facial paralysis and Horner's syndrome

        3. Cerebellar signs

        4. Ipsilateral facial hypesthesia for touch

        5. Contralateral body hypesthesia for pain and temperature

V. Treatment

    A. Anticoagulation with aspirin or other agents

        1. Anticoagulation has been demonstrated to decrease the frequency of transient ischemic attacks.

        2. Relative contraindications to anticoagulation include patient unreliability, diastolic blood pressure higher than 110 mmHg, blood dyscrasia, gastrointestinal bleeding, and severe liver disease.

    B. Consider extracranial vascular surgery if stenoses are identified.

    C. If head turning precipitates symptoms, a cervical collar is used.

VI. Natural course

    There is a 50 to 75% incidence of subsequent infarction in untreated patients with cerebrovascular insufficiency syndrome.

Multiple Sclerosis

I. Symptoms

    A. Vertigo

        1. Onset frequently in women during the third or fourth decade

        2. May persist for weeks or months and then subside

        3. Initial symptom in 5 to 15% of multiple sclerosis (M.S.) patients[10]

    B. Hearing loss and tinnitus: unusual but may occur as late symptoms

    C. Ask about other neurologic symptoms.

II. Signs
  A. Nystagmus
  B. Look for other neurologic signs.
III. Tests
  A. ABR is abnormal in 79% of patients who have brainstem symptoms.[11]
  B. Cerebrospinal fluid gamma globulin is elevated in 80 to 90% of patients during some time in the course of their disease.
IV. Treatment and prognosis
  A. M.S. runs a variable course.
  B. ACTH or steroids may be helpful during exacerbation.

REFERENCES

1. Clemis JD, Becker GW: Vestibular neuronitis. Otolaryngol Clin North Am 6:139, 1973

2. Brackmann DE, Anderson RG: Meniere's disease: treatment with the endolymphatic subarachnoid shunt, a review of 125 cases. Otolaryngol Head Neck Surg 88:174, 1980

3. Glasscock ME, Davis WE, Hughes GB, Jackson CG: Labyrinthectomy versus middle fossa vestibular nerve section in Meniere's disease: a critical evaluation of relief of vertigo. Ann Otol Rhinol Laryngol 89:318, 1980

4. Singleton GT, Karlan MS, Post KN, Bock DG: Perilymph fistulas: diagnostic criteria and therapy. Ann Otol Rhinol Laryngol 87:797, 1978

5. Wetmore SJ, Abramson M: Bullous myringitis with sensorineural hearing loss. Otolaryngol Head Neck Surg 87:66, 1979

6. Brandt T, Daroff RB: Physical therapy for benign paroxysmal positional vertigo. Arch Otolaryngol 106:484, 1980

7. Epley JM: Singular neurectomy: hypotympanotomy approach. Otolaryngol Head Neck Surg 88:304, 1980

8. Eggermont JJ, Don M, Brackmann DE: Electrocochleography and auditory brainstem electric responses in patients with pontine angle tumors. Ann Otol Rhinol Laryngol 89: suppl. 75:1, 1980

9. Burns RA: Basilar-vertebral artery insufficiency as cause of vertigo. Otolaryngol Clin North Am 6:287, 1973

10. Baloh RW: Dizziness, Hearing Loss and Tinnitus: The Essentials of Neurotology. p. 152. Davis, Philadelphia, 1984

11. Robinson K, Rudge P: Abnormalities of the auditory evoked potentials in patients with multiple sclerosis. Brain 100:19, 1977

12

Facial Nerve Paralysis

Stephen J. Wetmore

The diagnosis and treatment of peripheral facial paralysis, i.e., paralysis resulting from injuries peripheral to the brainstem, are dealt with in this chapter. Brainstem and peripheral facial paralyses usually present with unilateral paralysis involving all branches of the facial nerve. Brain lesions above the brainstem (supranuclear) usually result in sparing of forehead movement.

The most common cause of peripheral facial paralysis is idiopathic facial paralysis (Bell's palsy), a diagnosis made only after excluding other etiologies of the paralysis. The yearly incidence of Bell's palsy is 23/100,000.[1]

It is important not only to diagnose the etiology of the patient's facial paralysis but also to closely monitor the functional state of the facial nerve so that appropriate treatment can be instituted. The prognosis for recovery of facial nerve function depends largely on the severity of the injury. The prognosis significantly worsens when evidence of nerve degeneration is present regardless of the etiology. In order to institute proper treatment the functional state of the nerve and the location of the nerve injury must be determined.

FACIAL NERVE INJURY

I. Incidence
    A. Within temporal bone 95%[2]
        1. Bell's palsy 66.5%
        2. Trauma 13.5%
        3. Herpes zoster oticus 8.6%
        4. Otitis media 5.8%
        6. Neoplasia 5.5%
    B. Extratemporal 5%
        1. Trauma
        2. Parotid neoplasm
II. Pathophysiology
    A. Neuropraxia
        1. Reversible lesion
        2. Partial damming up of axioplasm
        3. Normal nerve excitability test
        4. Full recovery usually
    B. Axonotmesis

      1. Complete obstruction of axoplasmic flow in some nerve fibers
      2. Eventual degeneration of axons and myelin sheath from first node of Ranvier proximal to site of lesion to periphery
  C. Neurotmesis
      1. Involvement of whole nerve trunk
      2. Possible response of nerve to electrical stimulation for 48 to 72 hours post injury
      3. Complete degeneration of axons and myelin sheath (Wallerian degeneration)
      4. Nissl's degeneration of nerve cell body
  D. Regeneration
      1. Regeneration commences soon after degenerative process, provided there is no mechanical barrier.
      2. Schwann cells form cords of cells (tubules).
      3. Axons in proximal end of nerve proliferate and grow at 1 mm/day.
      4. Growing axon processes divide into many branches.
          a) Find their way into different cords
          b) Lead to sequelae of mass movement, facial spasm, and crocodile tears
III. Anatomy (Fig. 12-1)

    After traversing the internal auditory canal the facial nerve enters the narrow confines of the labyrinthine portion of the temporal bone. It makes an acute turn at the geniculate ganglion and then crosses the middle ear

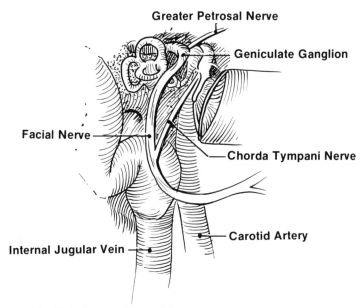

Fig. 12-1. Course of the facial nerve through the temporal bone.

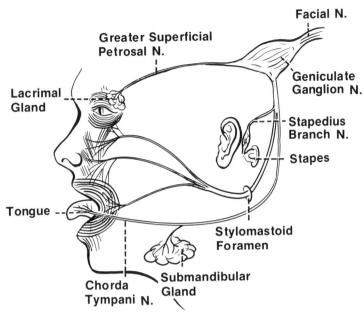

Fig. 12-2. Functional components of the facial nerve.

in a horizontal canal covered by a thin shell of bone. Next it curves inferiorly just deep to the posterior wall of the external auditory canal and exits through the stylomastoid foramen into the face.

IV. Diagnostic tests
   A. Site of lesion (topognostic) tests determine the location of the facial nerve injury by examining the function of the various branches of the nerve (Fig. 12-2).
      1. Geniculate ganglion
         a) Parasympathetic fibers pass through the geniculate ganglion en route to the lacrimal gland.
         b) Schirmer test for lacrimation (Fig. 12-3)
            (1) Most important site of lesion test
            (2) The end of a strip of filter paper is placed in the cul-de-sac of the lower eyelid for 5 minutes.
            (3) Tearing from both eyes is compared.
            (4) If tearing is diminished from the eye ipsilateral with the facial paralysis, it indicates that the site of injury is at or proximal to the geniculate ganglion. The best surgical approach to this portion of the facial nerve is a middle fossa craniotomy.
      2. Nerve to stapedius muscle
         a) Leaves the facial nerve along its vertical course in the mastoid bone
         b) Stapedius (acoustic) reflex

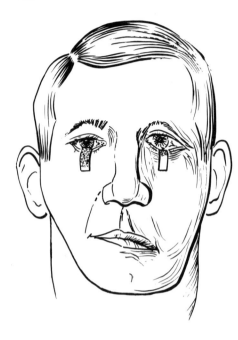

Fig. 12-3. Schirmer test. With facial nerve injury at or proximal to the geniculate ganglion, the eye on the paralyzed side of the face exhibits less tearing than the normal contralateral eye.

        (1) Reflex contraction of the muscle to loud sounds (70 to 85 dB).

        (2) Monitored with tympanometry

        (3) Not valid if conductive hearing loss present

  3. Chorda tympani

    a) Secretomotor fibers to submandibular and sublingual glands

    b) Taste fibers from anterior two-thirds of tongue

        (1) Taste testing

           i) Both sides of tongue tested with salt, sugar, and quinine

           ii) Not very accurate

        (2) Electrogustometry (electrical taste test)

           i) Small positive electrical current applied to the tongue produces a metallic or bitter taste

           ii) Compare electrical thresholds from both halves of tongue

           iii) It requires a subjective response.

           iv) There is large variability in response.

 B. Physiologic extent of nerve involvement

  1. Threshold facial nerve excitability test

    a) Stimulate various branches through skin with electrical stimuli in the 3 to 6 mA range

    b) Compare threshold at which movement occurs with the threshold of the opposite side.

    c) Test is not helpful during first 72 hours after injury, but thereafter it can differentiate neuropraxia from degeneration (elevated thresholds).

      d) Test is run daily for first week or two.
  2. Maximal nerve excitability test
      a) Similar to threshold test, but a current strong enough to produce maximal movement on the contralateral side of the face is used and then the degree of movement to the same stimulus on the paralyzed side is compared.
      b) Painful
  3. Electroneuronography (ENoG)[3]
      a) Similar in principle to the facial nerve excitability test, it uses a supramaximal electrical stimulus.
      b) Summating potential from the facial nerve is obtained from surface electrodes and recorded.
      c) Amplitude of summating potential is directly proportional to the number of functional nerve fibers.
      d) Comparing the amplitude from both sides of the face provides an objective record of the degree of degeneration.
      e) If amplitude of paralyzed side is less than that of noninvolved side, degeneration is likely to be taking place and surgical intervention is indicated.
      f) Equipment is relatively expensive and not as readily available as the standard hand-held facial nerve stimulator.
  4. Submandibular gland salivary flow[4]
      a) Cannulate submandibular ducts and measure salivary flow stimulated by a lemondrop. Collect three samples simultaneously from each side at 1-minute intervals.
      b) If salivary flow on paralyzed side is less than 25% of that on the contralateral side, there is a high likelihood that degeneration is occurring.
      c) Can predict degeneration immediately after injury, avoiding the 72-hour latent period for electrical testing. This allows earlier surgical intervention.
  5. Electromyography
      a) Needle is placed into muscle.
      b) Fibrillation potentials may be seen 14 to 21 days after injury if degeneration has occurred.
      c) Best used to show early signs of reinnervation after established degeneration

BELL'S PALSY (IDIOPATHIC FACIAL PARALYSIS)

I. Signs and symptoms
  A. Rapid onset of partial or complete hemifacial paralysis (minutes to hours)
  B. May have otalgia, facial pain, and/or facial numbness

C. May drool or complain of difficulty eating

D. Normal otologic examination

II. Diagnosis

    A. Audiogram: usually normal

    B. Mastoid x-ray film: helps rule out neoplasms

    C. Site of lesion tests: Schirmer test (see above) and stapedius reflex test (see above) most useful

    D. Test of facial nerve function (see above)

        1. If the patient has partial paralysis, monitor the degree of paralysis.

        2. The tests of facial nerve function are helpful in those patients who have complete paralysis because they differentiate neuropraxia from partial or complete facial nerve degeneration.

        3. Threshold or maximal nerve excitability tests are easiest to use.

        4. ENoG is more objective, but the necessary equipment is not as readily available.

        5. Submandibular salivary flow test may be a helpful prognostic test for patients seen within the first 48 hours after onset of complete paralysis.

III. Prognosis

    The prognosis depends on the degree of nerve injury.

    A. Partial paralysis: virtually 100% full recovery

    B. Complete paralysis but no signs of degeneration: 88% full recovery[4]

    C. Partial degeneration: 27% full recovery[4]

    D. Complete degeneration: incomplete recovery[4]

    E. Natural history: 63% with complete return[4]

    F. In patients who exhibit complete paralysis, the sooner the onset of facial movement, the better is the chance for complete recovery.[5]

        1. Among the group of patients who ultimately go on to full recovery, 50% note the beginning of movement within 2 weeks of paralysis, and the remainder within 4 weeks of paralysis.

        2. In the group of patients who ultimately exhibit poor recovery, 40% note onset of movement by 4 weeks, 50% by 8 weeks, and 100% by 12 weeks.

IV. Treatment

    A. Corticosteroids

        1. Controversy has raged over their efficacy in the treatment of Bell's palsy.

        2. Beneficial effect was proclaimed by Adour et al[6] in a large study done at the Kaiser-Permanente Clinic in Oakland, California.

            a) Treatment consisted of prednisone 40 mg/day for 4 days, tapering to 8 mg/day in 8 days.

            b) Comparison was made between 194 patients treated with prednisone and a historical control group of 110 untreated patients.

            c) Complete denervation occurred in 10% of the untreated group but in none of the treated group.

      d) Complete recovery of facial function occurred in 68% of the corticosteroid group but in only 43% of the untreated group.

      e) The criticisms of this study include the following:

        (1) Not double blind

        (2) Nonrandom distribution of patients

        (3) Historical controls

  3. A prospective randomized double-blind study by May et al[5] failed to show any benefits.

      a) Fifty-one patients seen within 2 days of onset of Bell's palsy were randomized to either steroids plus vitamins or to vitamins alone.

      b) Complete return of facial function occurred in 60% of the steroid group and in 65% of the control (vitamin) group.

  4. A large prospective randomized study by Wolf et al[7] showed minimal benefits of steroid therapy.

      a) A total of 239 patients seen within 5 days of onset of Bell's palsy were randomized either to a 17-day course of prednisone or to a nontreated control group.

      b) Complete recovery was noted in 88% of the steroid group and 80% of the controls. This difference was not statistically significant.

      c) The only statistically significant difference in outcome was for the complication of crocodile tearing, which was less frequent in the steroid group.

B. Surgical decompression for Bell's palsy.

  1. Controversial

  2. Probably indicated if degeneration occurs despite steroid therapy

TRAUMA

Temporal Bone Fracture (Basilar Skull Fracture)

I. Signs and symptoms

  A. *Longitudinal fracture* (along axis of temporal bone): 90% (Fig. 12-4). Results from force applied to temporoparietal region

    1. Bloody otorrhea secondary to laceration of external auditory canal and tympanic membrane

    2. Cerebrospinal fluid (CSF) otorrhea may occur

    3. Battle's sign: ecchymosis over mastoid skin

    4. Hearing loss secondary to blood in middle ear, tympanic membrane perforation, and/or ossicular disruption

    5. Facial paralysis in 10 to 18% of cases[8]

      a) Onset of paralysis often delayed

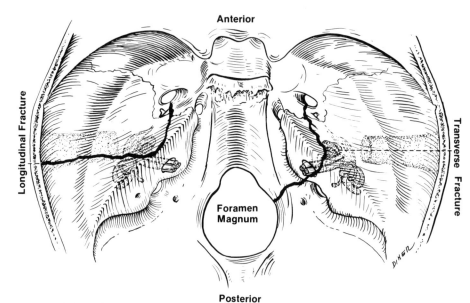

Fig. 12-4. View of the middle cranial fossa as seen from above. A longitudinal temporal bone fracture extends along the axis of the temporal bone and usually involves the external auditory canal. A transverse temporal bone fracture extends transversely across the main axis of the temporal bone and usually involves the internal auditory canal.

  b) If patient obtunded, try to elicit facial movement during physical examination using painful stimuli
 B. *Transverse fracture* (perpendicular to the longitudinal axis of the petrous portion of the temporal bone): 10% (Fig. 12-4); results from force applied to occipital region
  1. Hemotympanum
  2. Total unilateral sensorineural hearing loss in 50% of cases
  3. Facial paralysis in 38 to 50% of cases[8]
   a) Usually immediate and complete
   b) Try to elicit facial movement in comatose patient.
 II. Diagnosis
 A. Presence of facial weakness or paralysis
 B. Temporal bone tomogram or computed tomography (CT scan) to locate site of fracture
 C. Topognostic tests to determine site of nerve injury
 D. Electrical nerve testing to determine physiologic status of facial nerve
 III. Treatment
 A. If signs of nerve degeneration are present, surgical exploration and nerve repair are indicated as soon as possible if patient is stable from other major injuries.

B. Although patients with delayed onset of paralysis have a much better chance for complete recovery than those with immediate onset of paralysis, they are treated with surgical exploration if they show signs of nerve degeneration.

Facial Laceration with Facial Paralysis

I. Signs, symptoms, diagnosis
   A. Usually associated with deep lacerations in region of parotid gland or mastoid tip
   B. Check for facial nerve function prior to injecting the local anesthetic agent for any laceration that might involve the facial nerve trunk or its branches.
   C. Also look for a parotid duct laceration in any deep cheek laceration.
      1. Look for saliva coming from the parotid duct orifice while massaging the gland.
      2. Place lacrimal dilator into the duct orifice to see if it appears in the wound.
II. Treatment
   A. Primary nerve anastomosis using microsurgical techniques is considered.
      1. The operating room is the preferred setting.
      2. An electrical nerve stimulator may be helpful in locating the distal nerve branches if the repair is done within 48 hours of injury.
   B. Secondary repair is accomplished if associated injuries preclude primary anastomosis. If time permits, locating and tagging the nerve branches makes the second procedure easier.

Gunshot Wound to Face with Facial Paralysis

I. Signs, symptoms, and diagnosis
   A. Often massive soft tissue disruption is present.
   B. Check for facial nerve injury and parotid duct injury as with lacerations.
II. Treatment
   A. Often the associated injuries preclude primary nerve repair.
   B. Usually a nerve graft is needed if anastomosis is attempted as either an immediate or a delayed procedure.
   C. If direct nerve surgery cannot be performed, a fascial sling procedure can be done at a later date to pull up the drooping commissure of the lips, but the results are usually not as good as direct nerve surgery.

INFECTIONS

Acute Suppurative Otitis Media

I. Signs and symptoms
  A. Otalgia, an early sign of otitis media
  B. Otorrhea
    1. May occur hours or days after otalgia.
    2. Otalgia usually subsides when otorrhea begins.
  C. Possibly fever, anorexia, and malaise
  D. Hearing loss due to pus in middle ear
  E. Rapid onset of unilateral facial paralysis
II. Diagnosis
  A. Red, bulging tympanic membrane in early phase
  B. Otorrhea in later phase
  C. Facial paralysis, partial or complete
  D. Electrical nerve testing to check physiologic function
III. Treatment
  A. Antibiotics
  B. Myringotomy to ensure adequate drainage
  C. Steroids—controversial
  D. Surgery rarely needed, as most cases improve without developing nerve degeneration

Chronic Suppurative Otitis Media

I. Signs and symptoms
  A. Chronically draining ear
  B. Perforated tympanic membrane
  C. Rapid onset of facial paralysis
II. Diagnosis
  A. Topognostic and functional nerve tests
  B. Mastoid radiographs
III. Treatment
  A. Antibiotic ear drops plus systemic antibiotics are given.
  B. If nerve testing shows degeneration, treat by performing a facial nerve decompression (with mastoidectomy).

Herpes Zoster Oticus

I. Signs, symptoms, and diagnosis
  A. Presentation similar to that of Bell's palsy except for vesicles on the pinna

B. May exhibit sensorineural hearing loss
II. Treatment
   A. Treat like Bell's palsy
   B. Prognosis for recovery probably not as good as for Bell's palsy

NEOPLASMS

I. Types of neoplasms
   A. Within temporal bone
      1. Skin cancer of external auditory canal invading the mastoid
      2. Facial nerve neurilemmoma
      3. Acoustic neuroma: rarely produces facial paralysis before VIII and V nerve symptoms and signs
      4. Metastatic carcinoma
   B. Parotid neoplasms (malignant)
II. Signs and symptoms
   A. Gradual onset of paralysis (days to months)
   B. Twitching of face
   C. Otorrhea (ear canal tumors)
III. Treatment
   A. Surgery if possible
   B. Radiotherapy
   C. Chemotherapy

SUMMARY

I. Work-up of patient with facial nerve palsy
   A. Complete history and physical examination
   B. Site of lesion testing
   C. Physiologic state of nerve testing
   D. Possibly laboratory tests or x-ray studies depending on the etiology of the paralysis
II. Indicators of unfavorable prognosis
   A. Progression from partial to complete paralysis
   B. Loss of tearing
   C. Submandibular salivary flow less than 25%
   D. Elevated or absent response to electrical stimulation
III. Patients with an unfavorable prognosis should probably undergo surgical decompression.
IV. Alternatives for patients with no facial nerve function after more than 1 year
   A. Facial–hypoglossal anastomosis
   B. Fascial sling

REFERENCES

1. Hauser WA, Karnes WE, Annis J, Karland LT: Incidence and prognosis of Bell's palsy in the population of Rochester, Minnesota. Mayo Clinic Proc 46:258, 1971
2. Cawthorne T: Intratemporal facial palsy. Arch Otolaryngol 90:789, 1969
3. Fisch U: Maximal nerve excitability testing vs electroneuronography. Arch Otolaryngol 106:352, 1980
4. May M, Hardin WR, Sullivan J, Wette R: Natural history of Bell's palsy: the salivary flow test and other prognostic indicators. Laryngoscope 86:704, 1976
5. May M, Wette R, Hardin WB, Sullivan J: Use of steroids in Bell's palsy: a prospective controlled study. Laryngoscope 86:1111, 1976
6. Adour KK, Wingerd J, Bell DN, et al: Prednisone treatment for idiopathic facial paralysis (Bell's palsy). N Engl J Med 287:1268, 1972
7. Wolf SM, Wagner JH, Davidson S, Forsythe A: Treatment of Bell palsy with prednisone: a prospective, randomized study. Neurology (NY) 28:158, 1978
8. Harker LA, McCabe BF: Temporal bone fractures and facial nerve injury. Otolaryngol Clin North Am 7:425, 1974

13

Foreign Bodies

Robert W. Seibert _____

The critical physiologic importance of the upper airway, coupled with the propensity for children to accidentally or intentionally lodge objects in the numerous orifices and cavities of the head, make the subject of foreign bodies of major importance when discussing otolaryngologic emergencies.

Clinical presentation of a foreign body varies not only according to the anatomic site involved and the size, shape, and type of material of the foreign body, but according to other factors as well, such as the age of the patient and the degree of obstruction and inflammation elicited by the foreign body. Symptom severity may range from minimal to acutely life-threatening; a review of asphyxiation deaths in children revealed more than 700 deaths in 41 states over a 3-year period.[1] *The possibility of multiple foreign bodies must be considered, especially in the mentally retarded or psychotic patient.* Furthermore, the astute clinician always considers the possibility of a foreign body in a situation with an unusual or atypical clinical presentation, such as upper airway obstruction due to edema of the common tracheoesophageal wall, which may be caused by a chronic esophageal foreign body.

ANATOMIC SITE

Nose

The nose is the site of foreign bodies usually in children or retarded patients.
I. Signs and symptoms
  A. Rhinorrhea
    1. Unilateral discharge lasting several days to months
    2. Purulent: white to yellow-green pus, often tinged with dark blood
    3. Malodorous: often extremely foul-smelling discharge
    4. These three signs are strong evidence for a foreign body, especially in a child.
  B. Epistaxis
    1. Frank epistaxis uncommon
    2. Drainage usually blood-tinged only
II. Diagnosis
  A. Anterior rhinoscopy: requires good light and suction because exudate or blood may obscure foreign body.

217

    B. Radiographs are of limited value, as most foreign bodies are radiolucent.
III. Treatment
    A. Removal under controlled, atraumatic conditions in cooperative or anesthetized patient
    B. General anesthesia frequently required in children
    C. Equipment
        1. Light
        2. Suction
        3. Nasal speculum and forceps
    D. Systemic antibiotics to cover secondary rhinosinusitis

Nasopharynx

The nasopharynx is an uncommon site, but the situation may occur with posterior migration of a nasal foreign body.
  I. Signs and symptoms
    A. Rhinorrhea (as above)
    B. Posterior nasal drainage, mucoid to purulent
    C. Stridor, inspiratory
    D. Stertorous breathing (snoring)
 II. Diagnosis
    Lateral x-ray film of nasopharynx may be helpful.
III. Treatment
    Removal usually requires general anesthesia and removal by otolaryngologist.

Oropharynx/Hypopharynx

  I. Signs and symptoms
    A. Sharp objects such as fish bones and pins are prone to become lodged in palatine or lingual tonsils. Dental prostheses or teeth may become foreign bodies after head and neck trauma.
    B. In a young child, the history of an initial gagging episode may be missed.
    C. Pain—odynophagia (painful swallowing)
        1. Usually can localize side correctly
        2. Poor level (cephalad-caudad) localization
        3. May be referred to ear (otalgia)
    D. Dysphagia: difficulty swallowing, especially if foreign body is large
    E. Drooling: sign of severe swallowing dysfunction or pain in infant or young child
    F. Airway symptoms

    1. Partial obstruction of the hypopharyngeal airway produces dyspnea (air hunger) and stridor (noisy breathing) on inspiration.

    2. Intercostal, suprasternal, and substernal retractions are due to the increased negative intrapleural pressure and the use of the accessory respiratory muscles; they reflect increased work of breathing.

    3. Complete airway obstruction results in death or central nervous system (CNS) damage from hypoxemia within a few minutes.

II. Diagnosis

  A. Inspection

    Many foreign bodies are easily seen in oropharynx and tongue base.

  B. X-ray examination

    1. Thin bones and metal objects, especially nonferrous metals, may not be visible.

    2. Fish bones are usually cartilaginous and not usually seen on x-ray films.

III. Treatment

  A. In cooperative patient, removal with forceps under local or topical anesthesia.

  B. Removal under general anesthesia required in most children and uncooperative adults. *Note:* A hypopharyngeal foreign body may abruptly occlude the airway once relaxation under general anesthesia has occurred. Be prepared to do direct laryngoscopy and remove foreign body immediately.

  C. Complete obstruction: Emergent treatment is essential to save patient's life.

    1. If foreign body aspiration is known or strongly suspected, apply subdiaphragmatic pressure technique (Heimlich maneuver) (Fig. 13-1).[2]

    2. If patient is unconscious or obstruction is indicated by absence of air movement with continued thoracic wall motion, manage airway as follows:

      a) Position patient on back with neck hyperextended and mandible held forward, thus bringing tongue forward from posterior pharyngeal wall and assisting in clearing this portion of the airway (Fig. 13-2).

      b) If unsuccessful in establishing airway, endotracheal intubation via the oral route is done.

      c) If continued efforts are unsuccessful, emergency tracheotomy or cricothyrotomy may be necessary until definitive management of the foreign body can be done by an otolaryngologist.

IV. Complications

  A. Airway obstruction

  B. Perforating objects may lead to infection in adjacent tissue planes, retropharyngeal and lateral pharyngeal space. Clinician should be alert to late infectious complications.

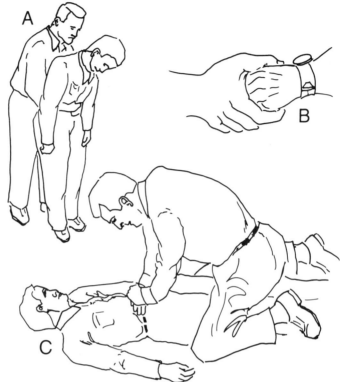

Fig. 13-1. (**A**) Rescuer approaches choking victim from behind, clasping hands (**B**) in front and applying sudden upward and inward thrust over epigastrium. (**C**) Choking victim is supine; rescuer kneels over victim, placing hands on epigastrium and applying thrust.

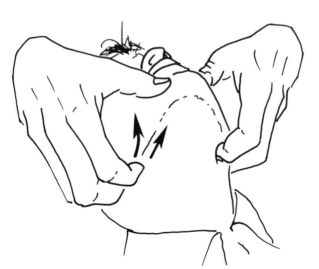

Fig. 13-2. Hold mandible forward to maximally open oropharyngeal airway.

Esophagus

I. Signs and symptoms
   A. Range from none to severe: dysphagia, drooling, stridor
   B. With *chronic* esophageal foreign bodies: secondary edema eventually compromising the tracheal airway (Fig. 13-3)
   C. Airway symptoms, especially *inspiratory* and *expiratory* stridor
II. Diagnosis
   A. Plain radiographs: Posteroanterior (PA) and lateral chest views
   B. Contrast esophagram usually not necessary[3]

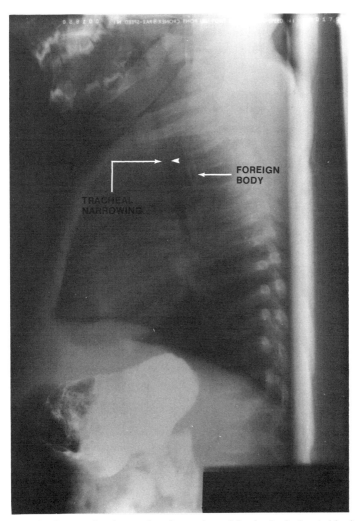

Fig. 13-3. Tracheal narrowing due to chronic esophageal foreign body (coated by barium).

C. Radiograph of neck and chest after swallowing small cotton ball soaked with barium which may stick to the foreign body and help localize it
III. Treatment
Removal via esophagoscopy, under general anesthesia in children and apprehensive adults

Larynx and Trachea

Potentially fatal due to complete obstruction of airway (see above). History of aspiration often absent.
I. Signs and symptoms
   A. Stridor
      1. Inspiratory: larynx
      2. Inspiratory and expiratory: tracheal and sometimes subglottic larynx
   B. Voice
      1. Hoarseness: glottic lesion
      2. Aphonia: may be complete obstruction. Requires emergency treatment: Heimlich maneuver, cricothyroidotomy, intubation, or emergency tracheotomy if no other alternative[4]
   C. Cough: nonspecific unless croup, which means subglottic lesion
II. Diagnosis
   A. Radiograph, soft tissue technique
   B. Lateral view of neck with videofluoroscopy
III. Treatment
Endoscopic removal under general anesthesia via direct laryngoscopy and/or bronchoscopy by experienced endoscopist. Be prepared to perform tracheostomy.

Bronchi

Obstruction from foreign body may range from none to partial or complete. Partial obstruction produces hyperinflation of lung distal to obstruction (obstructive emphysema) (Fig. 13-4). Complete obstruction produces atelectasis of distal lung (Fig. 13-5).
I. Signs and symptoms
   A. History of aspiration (e.g., choking, gagging) frequently absent
   B. Often latent period between aspiration and development of symptoms, i.e., cough, fever, wheezing, due to secondary infection
II. Diagnosis
   A. Unilateral wheezing: partially obstructing foreign body may produce prolonged expiration.
   B. Decreased or absent breath sounds signal complete obstruction.

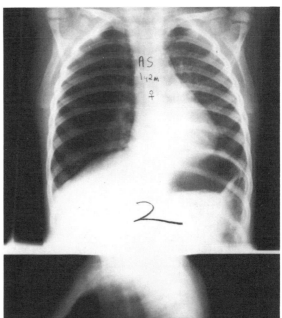

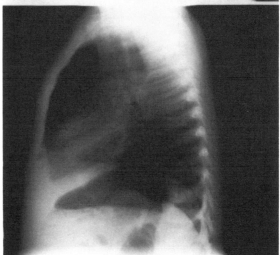

Fig. 13-4. Obstructive emphysema of the right lung due to a right main stem bronchial foreign body.

C. Signs of mediastinal shift toward side of lesion with atelectasis; away from side of lesion in obstructive emphysema
D. Radiographs
   1. Suspect radiolucent foreign body with atelectasis or recurrent, prolonged, or migratory pneumonia.
   2. Radiopaque foreign body is obvious.
   3. Inspiratory and expiratory chest x-ray films are obtained, looking for obstructive emphysema (Fig. 13-6).
   4. Right and left lateral decubitus: Look for absence of volume loss on the dependent side with partially obstructive foreign body; this is a good method in the uncooperative patient (Fig. 13-7).

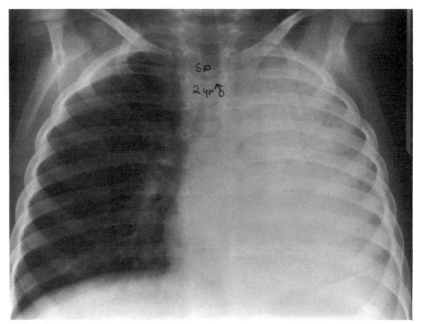

Fig. 13-5. Atelectasis of the left lung due to complete obstruction of the left main bronchus by a foreign body (bean).

     5. Videofluoroscopy may be done.
III. Treatment
    Bronchoscopy (rigid) under general anesthesia and removal of foreign body

Ear

The ear is a frequent site for foreign bodies in children.
I. Signs and symptoms
   A. Usually a small, smooth object (pebble, bead, popcorn kernel) which is difficult to grasp
   B. May be multiple and/or bilateral
   C. Severe discomfort: from live insects
   D. Often asymptomatic
   E. May cause secondary external otitis
   F. Occasionally bloody, purulent drainage
   G. Decreased hearing if ear canal is completely obstructed
II. Diagnosis
   A. Usually obvious on otoscopy
   B. Clear away exudate with suction or soft cotton-tipped applicator.

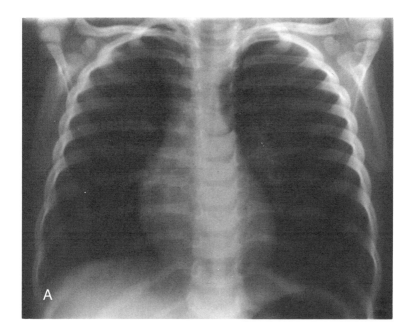

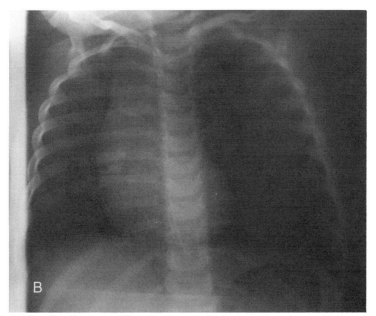

Fig. 13-6. (**A**) Routine chest x-ray film showing equal inflation of both lungs. (**B**) Expiratory chest x-ray film showing hyperinflation of the left lung due to partially obstructive left main stem bronchial foreign body.

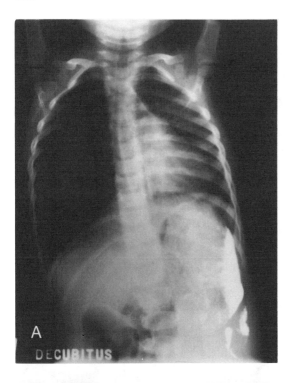

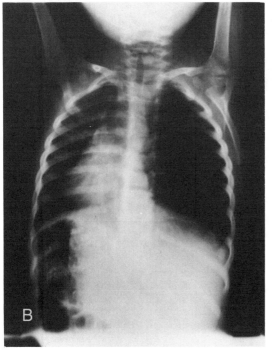

Fig. 13-7. (**A**) Left lateral decubitus x-ray film showing normal decreased volume of dependent left lung. (**B**) right lateral decubitus x-ray film, showing persistent overinflation of the right lung, indicating a partially obstructive right main stem bronchial foreign body.

III. Treatment
   A. Remove as gently as possible in awake patient. Bony external canal is exquisitely tender to touch.
   B. Ear canal can be irrigated if all of the following conditions are present:
      1. If space exists between the foreign body and the ear canal wall
      2. If the tympanic membrane is intact
      3. If the foreign body is not one that will expand when irrigated with water
   C. Instrument removal
      1. Forceps may be used to grasp object (difficult with a hard, smooth foreign body). A cerumen spoon may be used to gently manipulate foreign body out of ear.
      2. Heavy sedation or general anesthesia is frequently required in child.
      3. Avoid excessive manipulation in the uncooperative patient, as it may lead to external canal laceration or hematoma, tympanic membrane perforation, and even ossicular or inner ear trauma.[5]
      4. Refer to otolaryngologist if chances for atraumatic removal appear limited.

REFERENCES

1. Harris CS, Baker SP, Smith GA, et al: Childhood asphyxiation by food: a national analysis and overview. JAMA 251:2231, 1984
2. Heimlich HJ: First aid for choking children: back blows and chest thrusts cause complications and death. Pediatrics 70:120, 1982
3. Turtz MG, Stool SE: Foreign bodies of the pharynx and esophagus. In Bluestone CD, Stool SE (eds): Pediatric Otolaryngology. WB Saunders, Philadelphia, 1983
4. Tucker JA: Obstruction of the major pediatric airway. Otolaryngol Clin North Am 12:329, 1979
5. Broennie AM, Gewitz MH, Handler SD, et al: Illustrated techniques of pediatric emergency procedures. In Fleisher G, Ludwig S (eds): Textbook of Pediatric Emergency Medicine. Williams & Wilkins, Baltimore, 1984

14

Caustic Ingestions

Robert W. Seibert _____

Accidentally or intentionally ingested caustic agents result in significant morbidity and mortality. An estimated 5,000 to 8,000 cases of lye ingestion occur each year in children.[1] While in children these incidents are predominantly accidental, in teenagers and adults ingestion of such corrosive agents is usually a suicide attempt.

The responsible agents fall into three categories.

1. *Detergents and cleaners* (e.g., soaps, bleaches, and ammonia compounds). These agents cause mild to moderate gastrointestinal irritation with symptoms such as nausea, vomiting, and diarrhea. Mucosal ulceration usually does not occur except with concentrated ammonia solutions.[2] Esophageal injury and stricture formation after ingestion of household bleach has been reported rarely.

2. *Alkali and alkaline products* (e.g., drain and toilet bowl cleaners). These are strong, caustic agents capable of producing rapid and severe gastrointestinal injury.

3. *Acidic products* (e.g., hydrochloric, nitric, and sulfuric acids). These products cause gastric and esophageal injury.

GENERAL PRINCIPLES OF MANAGEMENT

I. As always, prevention is better than treatment. "Poison proofing" consists of the following measures.[2]
   A. Store agent out of sight and reach of children.
   B. Keep agents in original containers, never in bottles or food containers.
   C. Secure storage areas by safety latches or locks.
   D. Purchase the least toxic products in the smallest amounts necessary for the job.
   E. Buy agents in child-resistant containers.
   F. After a product has been used return it immediately to the storage area.
   G. Be especially careful when home routine is changed, such as when visiting during holidays.
II. Any child who has been found with an open container of a caustic substance should be assumed to have ingested it and sustained a caustic injury until proved otherwise. This is true even in the presence of a normal oral

and oropharyngeal examination, as 10 to 15% of esophageal burns have
no associated oropharyngeal injury.[3]

III. Telephone advice
   A. Immediate treatment at home includes giving the patient large amounts
      of water to drink to dilute the ingested substance. Milk or antacids
      may be used in alkaline ingestions.
   B. Do *not* induce vomiting. Gastric lavage or emetics are contraindicated
      because they may cause further damage.[2]
   C. Attempting to neutralize the pH of the ingested substance by giving a
      solution of the opposite pH is ineffective and may produce more injury
      by the exothermic chemical reaction that may result.
   D. Transport patient immediately to the hospital.

ALKALINE BURNS

I. Agents
   Substances that produce alkaline burns include drain and toilet cleaners
   that contain strong alkalis, especially sodium hydroxide. They are found
   in solid (crystalline) and liquid forms, the latter associated with much
   greater risk of severe esophageal and gastric burns. Solids are usually
   spit out by a child before large amounts are ingested.

II. Mechanism of injury
   Injury is produced by precipitation of tissue protein and saponification
   of fats, producing penetrating burns of the gastrointestinal tract. The
   depth of a burn varies from mucosal to transmural, depending on the
   form, concentration, and duration of contact of the ingested substance.
   Liquid alkalis produce the greatest injuries, including transmural necrosis
   of the stomach and small bowel.[4] Solid agents usually do not reach the
   stomach owing to gastroesophageal sphincter spasm. Regurgitation of the
   material then occurs.

III. Signs and symptoms
   A. Burning sensation in the mouth and chest (esophagus) is usual.
   B. Dysphagia is frequent and combined with increased salivation leads
      to drooling. Dysphagia is due both to esophageal spasm, pain, and
      inflammatory edema.
   C. Vomiting of bloody material may occur.
   D. Stridor may be seen due to laryngeal swelling secondary to aspiration
      which results from swallowing dysfunction or may be simply due to
      a severe hypopharyngeal burn.
   E. The mouth or pharynx may vary in appearance from normal to the
      presence of whitish patches or inflamed and ulcerated mucosa.
   F. If there are two or more symptoms—vomiting, drooling, or stridor—
      there is a 50% chance of an associated esophageal burn.[5]

G. Esophageal perforation, mediastinitis, and/or shock and subsequent cardiovascular collapse may occur with a severe injury.

H. Although there is anywhere from a 25 to 70% chance that oropharyngeal burns are not accompanied by esophageal injury,[6] there is also a 15% chance that there is esophageal injury and no concomitant oropharyngeal burns.

IV. Diagnosis

A. Esophagoscopy under general anesthesia by an experienced endoscopist is done within 12 to 24 hours of the ingestion in all known *or* suspected cases. This is done to definitively establish the presence or absence of esophageal and/or gastric injury.[5] It cannot be overemphasized that significant esophageal injury leading to perforation or stricture formation may exist without an oropharyngeal burn. Therefore, esophagoscopy is mandatory unless contraindicated by impending airway obstruction or evidence of esophageal perforation such as mediastinitis or shock.

B. If esophagoscopy is not possible, certain radiographic features are extremely helpful in diagnosing esophageal injury.[7]

1. For mild injury, a contrast esophagram may show delayed passage of contrast or edematous esophageal mucosal folds and linear ulceration.

2. In severe injury, findings may include a rigid, narrowed esophagus, a dilated atonic esophagus, or an esophagus showing increased irritability and uncoordinated peristaltic activity.

V. Management in children

A. The following protocol for management of acute alkaline burns in children (within first 48 hours) has been suggested.[5]

1. Obtain history and identify caustic agent.

2. Place patient on "nothing by mouth."

3. Start an intravenous line; type and crossmatch blood.

4. Notify otolaryngology and pediatric surgery services.

5. Obtain permission for esophagoscopy.

6. Obtain hematocrit value and urinalysis.

7. Check heart and lungs for clearance for general anesthesia.

8. Obtain x-ray film on admission.

9. Perform esophagoscopy, ideally within 12 hours after ingestion; may be done up to 48 hours after ingestion. After this time the increased risk of perforation of a weakened esophageal wall precludes instrumentation.

10. Obtain contrast esophagram with videofluoroscopy within 24 hours, if possible. An esophagram is useful for evaluating the esophagus distal to the level of the most proximal circumferential burn, which should be the most distal point of direct visualization at esophagoscopy. After 48 hours, a contrast esophagram may be the only diagnostic tool to indicate severe esophageal injury.

Although expensive, the contrast agent metrizamide (Amipaque) is well tolerated even in the presence of aspiration or esophageal perforation. Most patients, especially children, refuse to swallow so that the agent must be introduced into the pharynx or proximal esophagus via a small caliber tube passed through the nose. For follow-up studies (see below) barium may be used.

   B. No esophageal injury

      1. Care for mouth burn with topical antibiotic ointment and local hygiene.

      2. Discharge patient when healing of the oral burns has progressed sufficiently to allow eating.

      3. Patient returns for outpatient follow-up.

         a) No esophageal symptoms: return 1 year

         b) Suggestive esophageal symptoms: videofluoroscopy with esophagram and dilation, as indicated

   C. Injured esophagus

      1. Administer steroids immediately (must be within 48 hours); prednisone (or equivalent) 3 to 5 mg/kg/day for 3 weeks

      2. Give antibiotics: cephalexin (Keflex) for 10 days.

      3. Hydrate with intravenous fluids until patient can swallow saliva, which usually occurs within 48 hours.

      4. Allow clear liquid diet when patient is able to swallow; advance to soft diet as tolerated.

      5. Repeat esophageal videofluoroscopy 3 weeks after burn.

         a) If significant stricture, stop steroids and begin dilatation.

         b) If no stricture, stop steroids and follow monthly as outpatient for 1 year.

VI. Management in adults

   A. Ingestion of alkaline agents in adults is much less common than in children but may be more serious because larger quantities are ingested. These are usually suicide attempts.

   B. If only a small amount of caustic agent is ingested, the management outlined above is adequate.

   C. If a large quantity is ingested and there are severe burns of the oral cavity and hypopharynx, it is likely that the esophagus and larynx have severe burns. The following are considered in the management of these cases:

      1. Perform tracheotomy if the patient has airway distress.

      2. Have patient be seen by thoracic and/or general surgeons to consider a total esophagectomy with either a stomach pull-up or a colon interposition. With severe necrosis of the esophagus, perforation and major blood vessel rupture are almost imminent.

VII. Healing

   A. Healing occurs in three phases:

      1. Acute necrosis, during days 1 to 4

2. Ulceration–granulation, days 5 to 15 (esophageal wall weakest during this period)
3. Cicatrization and stricture formation, beginning during the third and fourth weeks
   B. With final healing there is frequently dysphagia (due to esophageal strictures) and/or hiatal hernia (due to shortening of the esophagus).

ACIDIC BURNS

I. Agents
   The mineral acids, e.g., hydrochloric acid, nitric acid, and sulfuric acid, are the most commonly ingested.
II. Mechanism of injury
   Acidic agents cause coagulation necrosis of tissue which may prevent deep penetration of the burn into the esophageal wall. The stomach and duodenum are more likely to be injured than the esophagus. With healing, narrowing of the gastric antrum and consequent gastric outlet obstruction may occur.
III. Signs and symptoms
   A. Frequently, a burning sensation in the mouth, chest, and abdomen
   B. Commonly, dysphagia and hematemesis
   C. Possible abdominal pain and acute abdominal signs
   D. Examination of the mouth and oropharynx may reveal inflamed mucosa with whitish areas and/or ulceration.
IV. Management
   A. Encourage patient to drink water but do *not* use alkalizing solution such as sodium bicarbonate in an attempt to neutralize the agent.
   B. Do *not* lavage stomach or induce vomiting.
   C. Treat any cutaneous burns of the mouth and face with topical antibiotics; local débridement and cleaning are done as indicated.
   D. Hospitalize the patient immediately, provide general supportive care, and observe closely for signs of gastric perforation—in which case a laparotomy is indicated.
   E. Prophylactic antibiotics and steroids are not indicated.
   F. Perform upper gastrointestinal series 3 to 6 weeks postingestion.
   G. Watch for a possible complication of gastric injury, outlet obstruction with vomiting due to prepyloric scarring and stenosis. General surgical consultation and treatment are indicated for this condition.

REFERENCES

1. Leape LL, Ashcraft KW, Scarpelli DG, Holder TM: Hazard to health: liquid lye. N Engl J Med 284:578, 1971
2. McGuigon MA: Treatment of poisoning. Clin Symp 36:3, 1984

3. Borja AR, Randell HT, Thomas TV, Johnson W: Lye injuries of the esophagus—analysis of ninety cases of lye ingestion. J Thorac Cardiovasc Surg 57:533, 1969
4. Crain EF, Gershel JC, Mezey AP: Caustic ingestions—symptoms as predictors of esophageal injury. Am J Dis Child 138:863, 1984
5. Haller JA Jr: Corrosive stricture of the esophagus. p. 472. In Mavitch MM, Welch KJ, Benson CO (eds): Pediatric Surgery. 3rd Ed. Vol. 1. Year Book, Chicago, 1979
6. Buntain WL, Cain WC: Caustic injuries to the esophagus: a pediatric overview. South Med J 75:590, 1981
7. Franken EA: Caustic damage to the gastrointestinal tract: roentgen features. Am J Roent 188:77, 1973

15

Oral Cavity Emergencies

Stephen J. Wetmore
Hassan Bashiri

DENTAL EMERGENCIES

Infection

Pericoronitis

Pericoronitis is usually seen surrounding a partially erupted mandibular molar. The third molar is especially susceptible because the soft tissue flap usually present over its occlusal surface traps food debris and bacteria. This flap can be traumatized during mastication, further inflaming the tissue.

I. Signs and symptoms
   A. Red and edematous tissue, often in the third molar region
   B. Pain
   C. Adjacent soft tissue irritation
   D. Trismus
   E. Difficulty swallowing
   F. Chills, fever, general malaise, constipation
   G. Foul-smelling breath
   H. Enlarged, tender cervical lymph nodes
II. Treatment
   A. Irrigate with normal saline solution.
   B. Initiate antibiotic therapy, e.g., penicillin or erythromycin.
   C. Administer analgesics, e.g., acetaminophen with codeine.
   D. Refer to a dentist, who may remove the excess tissue overlying the tooth or consider extraction of the tooth after symptoms have subsided if it is growing outside the dental arch or if there is not enough room for it to erupt. Most third molars do not need extraction.

Acute Pulpitis

The dental pulp located in the center of the tooth is composed of delicate connective tissue containing tiny blood vessels, lymphatics, and nerves. Acute pulpitis usually occurs in a tooth with a large carious lesion or with a restoration around which recurrent caries have developed.

I. Signs and symptoms
   A. Pain
      1. Elicited by hot or cold food
      2. Persists after the stimulus has been removed
      3. May be severe and lancinating, especially if the entrance to the diseased pulp is narrow, resulting in buildup of pressure from the development of a pulp abscess
      4. May be dull and throbbing if a large cavity is present, precluding the buildup of pressure in the pulp chamber
   B. The tooth is not particularly sensitive to percussion unless the inflammation extends beyond the pulp tissue and into the root apex.

II. Treatment
   A. Analgesics
   B. Antibiotics
   C. Refer to a dentist, who usually treats by opening the pulp chambers to remove the pus. Subsequent root canal therapy and placement of a crown is often necessary, but tooth extraction is often unnecessary.

Periapical Abscess

I. Etiology

The etiology of periapical abscess is an infection of the apex of the tooth root, usually caused by decay of the tooth allowing infection to spread along the root canal of the tooth to the apex area. This condition may also result from a chronic periodontal abscess that gradually goes deep to the apex area and into the pulp. The involved teeth are usually nonvital, i.e., the pulp tissue has necrosed.

II. Signs and symptoms
   A. Extremely painful tooth
   B. Tooth sometimes slightly extended from its socket
   C. Possible intraoral swelling close to the involved tooth
   D. In a chronic abscess, sometimes an intraoral or extraoral fistula
   E. With an acute periapical abscess, slight thickening of the periodontal membrane may be the only radiologic abnormality; with a chronic abscess, a round radiolucency at the apex of the involved tooth is usually present.

III. Treatment
   A. Antibiotic therapy, e.g., penicillin or erythromycin.
   B. Analgesics
   C. Refer to a dentist for apicectomy and root canal therapy or extraction of involved tooth depending on stage and severity of infection.

Acute Osteomyelitis of Mandible or Maxilla

Acute osteomyelitis is an infection of the bone and bone marrow that may either result from a periapical abscess or be secondary to a fracture of the jaw.

I. Signs and symptoms
   A. Intense pain over the diseased portion of the jaw
   B. Swelling of the adjacent soft tissue
   C. Pus draining from around the gingiva of the teeth
   D. Teeth sometimes elevated and loose
   E. Paresthesias or anesthesia of the lip possible
   F. Irregular areas of densities and lucencies of the bone on x-ray films
II. Treatment
   A. Systemic antibiotics for at least 30 days, e.g., penicillin
   B. Treatment of diseased teeth; usually involves extraction
   C. Débridement of bone sequestra sometimes necessary

Soft Tissue Abscess of Dental Origin

Infections of dental origin may spread to the soft tissues of the face and neck either by direct extension, e.g., from a periapical abscess that has eroded through the cortex of the mandible or maxilla, or by lymphatogenous spread of an odontogenic infection of any type.

I. Signs and symptoms
   A. Pain, swelling, and tenderness of the involved soft tissue
   B. Usually systemic findings, e.g., fever and leukocytosis
II. Location of abscess and treatment
   Location of the abscess depends on which tooth is infected. It is usually necessary to incise and drain (I & D) the abscess as well as to treat the infected tooth, which often necessitates tooth extraction.
   A. Buccinator space
      1. Cheek swelling
      2. Maxillary molar or premolars involved
      3. Usually can I & D intraorally
   B. Infratemporal fossa
      1. Swelling inferior to zygomatic arch
      2. Maxillary second and third molars involved
      3. I & D intraorally
   C. Sublingual space
      1. Swelling in floor of mouth may progress to Ludwig's angina (see Ch. 6).
      2. Mandibular incisors, canines, premolars, or sometimes first molars
      3. I & D intraorally
   D. Submandibular triangle

    1. Differentiate from submandibular gland sialadenitis and submandibular triangle lymphadenitis (see Ch. 7).
    2. Mandibular molar roots extend below the insertion of the mylohyoid muscle and may result in submandibular triangle rather than floor of mouth infection. If the infection progresses, both anatomic areas may be involved in what is then called Ludwig's angina (see Ch. 6).
    3. I & D through the submandibular triangle.
  E. Parapharyngeal space
    1. Swelling of the upper neck below the angle of the mandible with deviation of the lateral oropharyngeal wall toward the midline
    2. Mandibular molars involved
    3. This is a deep neck abscess which should be approached through a neck incision.
  F. Maxillary sinusitis
    1. Toothache plus tenderness to palpation and percussion over the maxillary sinus; foul-smelling purulent rhinorrhea may be present.
    2. The roots of the maxillary molars and premolars often extend into the maxillary sinus with only a thin shell of bone separating the roots from the mucosa of the sinus.
    3. Caldwell-Luc and nasoantral windows are often necessary. After extracting the infected tooth, an oroantral fistula is often present that requires surgical closure.

Trauma

Fractured Tooth

  I. Types of fracture
    A. Enamel: Tooth looks normal except for a small piece of enamel chipped off.
    B. Enamel and dentin: Can see yellow color of tooth, and the tooth is somewhat sensitive.
    C. Enamel, dentin, and pulp: Can see redness of pulp chamber and sometimes bleeding from pulp canal; very sensitive.
  II. Treatment
    Refer to a dentist; if pulp chamber is exposed, root canal therapy is necessary to save the tooth.

Loose Tooth

Splint the loose tooth by wiring it with No. 26 wire to an adjoining stable tooth, or send patient to dentist.

Displaced Tooth

Reposition tooth with finger pressure into correct position and then wire to a stable adjoining tooth.

Avulsed Tooth

Gently clean the tooth and replace into its socket as soon as possible. The shorter the period that the tooth is out of its socket, the greater the success rate for reimplantation. The tooth will need to be wired or splinted into place and will probably need root canal therapy if it stays in place. Antibiotics recommended.

Mandible Fracture

I. Alveolar ridge fractures
  A. Signs and symptoms
    1. Appear as two or three adjacent loose and usually displaced teeth
    2. May have more than one alveolar ridge fracture and may have other mandible or maxillary fractures
  B. Treatment
    1. Anesthetize the injured area.
    2. Reduce the fractured segment(s).
    3. Use an arch bar or an acrylic splint to attach the teeth to adjacent stable teeth.
II. Other types of mandible and maxillary fractures (see Ch. 2)

TEMPOROMANDIBULAR JOINT PROBLEMS

Dislocated Mandible

I. Signs and symptoms
  A. Sudden locking of jaws in the wide open position
    1. Mouth cannot be closed.
    2. Eating and talking are difficult.
  B. Usually occurs as a result of opening the mouth too widely, such as when yawning and during dental treatment
  C. Head of the condyle moves anterior to the articular condyle and cannot be returned to the glenoid fossa voluntarily (Fig. 15-1).
  D. Spasmodic contraction of the temporalis, lateral pterygoid, and masseter muscles occurs.

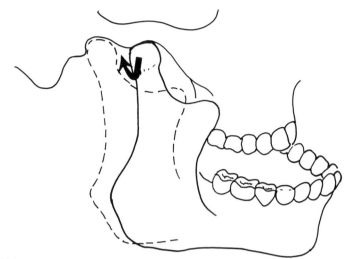

Fig. 15-1. Dislocated mandible. Arrow shows direction through which the condyle must be maneuvered to return it to the glenoid fossa.

II. Treatment
   A. Relaxation of spasmodically contracted muscles
      1. Analgesics, such as meperidine hydrochloride (Demerol), 50 to 75 mg I.M.
      2. Muscle relaxants, e.g., intravenous diazepam in a carefully titrated dose of 5 to 10 mg
      3. Injection of 1 to 2 ml of 1% lidocaine with 1:100,000 epinephrine into each joint space: usually relocates jaw immediately
      4. General anesthesia occasionally necessary
   B. After the muscles relax using one or more of the above methods, manual reduction can usually be accomplished by the physician placing thumbs in the mandibular molar region lateral to the teeth and applying downward and posterior pressure while at the same time placing a finger on the patient's neck and applying upward motion to the chin (Fig. 15-2).
   C. After reducing the dislocation, caution the patient to avoid opening his jaw widely for several weeks.
   D. For patients who develop recurrent dislocation of the mandible, elective surgical treatment may be necessary.

Temporomandibular Joint Pain Dysfunction Syndrome

I. Etiology[1]
   A. Masticatory muscle spasm as a result of overextension, overcontraction, or fatigue

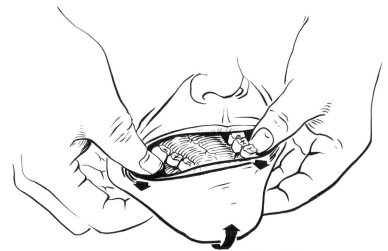

Fig. 15-2. Relocation of dislocated mandible.

1. Muscle overextension may result from dental restorations or prosthetic appliances which encroach on the space between the upper and lower teeth.
2. Muscle overcontraction may result from overclosure of the dental arches due to bilateral loss of posterior teeth or continued resorption of alveolar bone from under dentures.
3. Muscle fatigue is caused by grinding or clenching the teeth.
B. Malocclusion often occurs from spasm of masticatory muscles.
C. Trauma to the jaws is the inciting event in some patients.
D. A psychosomatic component is often present.
   1. A history of bruxism (teeth grinding) especially at night can often be elicited.
   2. Other psychophysiologic diseases such as peptic ulcers and migraine headaches occur frequently in these patients.
II. Signs and symptoms
   A. Mostly female patients, usually below age 40
   B. Pain
      1. Usually unilateral
      2. Main complaint: earache—chronic dull ache localized to the ear or the preauricular area
      3. Sometimes radiates to temporal area, angle of mandible, or neck
   C. Muscle tenderness usually present in the lateral pterygoid, temporalis, or masseter muscle
   D. Clicking or popping noise often present in temporomandibular joint
   E. Uneven opening motion of the mandible with lateral deviation of the mandible
   F. Malocclusion often

G. If edentulous, often has old or poor-fitting dentures

H. Absence of tenderness in the temporomandibular joint itself and absence of radiologic abnormalities of the joint

III. Treatment

Multiple approaches have been used.

A. Liquid diet for several days

B. Relaxation of the muscles of mastication with warm compresses and muscle relaxants plus mild analgesics

C. Readjustment of the occlusion
1. Clear plastic acrylic splints designed by a prosthodontist or dentist with expertise in this area are recommended.
2. The edentulous patient may need new dentures or relining of his old ones.
3. Patients with several missing teeth often need removable partial dentures or crown and bridge work.
4. Adjustment of the occlusion by grinding away the teeth is avoided.

D. Treatment of any underlying psychosocial problems

ORAL CAVITY EMERGENCIES

Trauma

Lacerations

See Chapter 2.

Food Burns

I. Signs and symptoms
A. Can affect any portion of the oral cavity
B. Usually very painful for a day or two after actual burn occurred
C. Visible membrane sometimes formed over burned mucosa

II. Treatment
A. Irrigation with a baking soda solution, 1.5 cc per cup of water
B. Analgesic
1. Pain medication
2. Viscous lidocaine 2%: rinse mouth with 5 ml as needed for pain

Caustic Ingestion

See Chapter 14.

Electrical Burns

I. Signs and symptoms
   A. In young children who bite on electrical cords
   B. Injury usually in the oral commissure
   C. Often more extensive than what appears on the skin surface, also involving the subcutaneous tissues, muscle, and underlying mucosa
   D. Lesions of varying size
   E. Often a full thickness burn with a centrally depressed white or yellow crater surrounded by a zone of slightly elevated pale gray tissue
      1. Edema occurs within hours.
      2. An eschar forms and then sloughs in 2 to 3 weeks.
II. Treatment
   A. Local wound care including an antibiotic ointment
   B. Oral antibiotics: penicillin recommended
   C. Some of the burns may not look serious, but caution is taken to prevent facial deformity caused by contracture of the oral and perioral tissues, particularly at the commissure. A removable acrylic commissure expanding appliance[2] can be fabricated by a prosthodontist and fitted to the patient within a week after the burn. This appliance helps prevent scar tissue contracture of the lips.

Ulcerations

Aphthous Ulcers (Canker Sores)

I. Etiology
   A. A pleomorphic L-form of the alpha-hemolytic *Streptococcus sanguis* may be the causative agent.[3]
   B. Precipitating factors for recurrent ulcers
      1. Local trauma such as self-inflicted bites, dental procedures
      2. Endocrine conditions
         a) Greatest incidence during premenstrual period
         b) Remission often seen during pregnancy with recurrence following parturition
      3. Psychological factors: stress may precipitate ulcer appearance
      4. Allergy: food or drug allergies
II. Signs and symptoms
   A. Occur slightly more frequently in women than men
   B. Onset of the disease usually between ages 10 and 30 years
   C. Frequency of aphthae considerably variable
   D. Begins as single or multiple superficial erosions covered by a gray membrane
      1. Well-circumscribed margin surrounded by an erythematous halo

      2. No vesicle formation during development of the ulcer

      3. Vary in size from 2 to 10 mm in diameter

  E. Occur on oral mucosa that is *not* attached to periosteum

  F. Painful

  G. Number of aphthae per outbreak may vary but usually fewer than six.

  H. Ulcers persist 7 to 14 days and then usually heal without scarring.

III. Treatment

  No currently available treatment is dramatically helpful.

  A. Tetracycline suspension (250 mg/5 ml) held in the mouth for 2 minutes and then swallowed produces a statistically significant response rate in terms of ulcer duration, size, and pain when administered four times per day for 1 week.[4]

  B. Steroid paste (0.1% triamcinolone acetonide dental paste) may be helpful.

  C. Chemical cautery may help relieve pain.

Herpes Simplex Infections

I. Primary herpetic stomatitis

  A. Etiology

    1. Herpes simplex virus

    2. Virus recovered from saliva

  B. Signs and symptoms

    1. In children and young adults

    2. Prodrome of fever, irritability, headache, malaise, odynophagia, and cervical adenopathy

    3. Within a few days the mouth becomes painful and the gingiva intensely inflamed; drooling, dysphagia, and dehydration can occur.

    4. Yellow vesicles 1 to 10 mm occur anywhere in the oral cavity; often multiple sites are involved simultaneously.

    5. After rupture of the vesicles, a shallow ulcer forms, covered by a gray membrane and surrounded by erythema.

    6. Ulcers are very painful.

    7. Spontaneous healing occurs in 7 to 14 days.

  C. Diagnosis

    1. Reliably made by examining a Papanicolaou smear using fresh scrapings from the base of the vesicles and identifying the characteristic histologic features

    2. Viral cultures impractical, though reliable

  D. Treatment

    1. Symptomatic therapy

    2. Acyclovir may prove to be beneficial especially in immunosuppressed patients but must be used early.

II. Secondary (recurrent) herpes labialis and stomatitis

  A. Etiology

1. Herpes virus appear to lie dormant within regional nerve ganglia and when reactivated spread along nerves to sites on the oral mucosa and skin.
   2. Precipitating factors appear to be trauma, menstruation, pregnancy, upper respiratory infection, emotional stress, fatigue, and exposure to ultraviolet light.
   B. Signs and symptoms
   1. Herpes labialis
      a) Tiny vesicles occur in clusters and present on the lips near the vermilion–cutaneous junction.
      b) The vesicles may be only 1 mm in size but often coalesce and are surrounded by erythema.
      c) After the vesicles rupture a brown crust covers the lesion.
   2. Herpes stomatitis
      a) The intraoral lesions usually occur on epithelium that is tightly bound to periosteum, in contrast to aphthous ulcers which usually occur on loosely bound mucosa.
      b) Vesicles are not often seen in the mouth; instead, an ulcer surrounded by erythema and covered by a gray membrane occurs.
   3. Lesions are preceded by a burning sensation where vesicles later erupt.
   4. Pain is variable in degree.
   5. Healing occurs in 7 to 10 days without scarring.
   C. Diagnosis
   Cytologic examination as mentioned under primary herpetic simplex infection can be performed.
   D. Treatment
   1. Acyclovir 5% in propylene glycol base has been shown to decrease the duration of vesiculation and to decrease the time until complete healing occurs.[5] Treatment begins during the prodrome of a "burning sensation." Acyclovir cream is applied 5 times per day for 5 days.
   2. Systemic acyclovir is effective in preventing recurrent herpes simplex infections in immunodeficient patients.[6]

Herpangina

I. Etiology
   A. Coxsackie group A virus
   B. Incubation period 3 to 5 days
   C. Commonly multiple cases in single household
II. Signs and symptoms
   A. Occurs mainly in young children
   B. Frequently occurs in sporadic outbreaks especially in summer

    C. Prodrome is a sore throat, fever, headache, and sometimes vomiting, prostration, and abdominal pain.

    D. Small ulcers appear on a gray base with surrounding erythema.

    E. Ulcers are located on the tonsillar pillars, hard and soft palate, and tongue.

    F. Pain often is not severe.

III. Treatment and sequelae

    A. Self-limiting disease without specific treatment

       1. Analgesics

       2. Topical anesthetics

       3. Bland diet

       4. Hydration

    B. Occasionally parotitis or meningitis

Behçet's Syndrome

  I. Etiology

    Uncertain

 II. Signs and symptoms

    A. Syndrome of oral and genital ulcerations, ocular lesions, and skin lesions

    B. Mainly in male patients between age 10 and 30 years

    C. Oral lesions: painful and similar in appearance to aphthous ulcers

    D. Genital ulcers: small and appear on the scrotum, root of the penis, and labia majora

    E. Ocular lesions: from conjunctivitis to uveitis

    F. Skin lesions: small pustules or papules on the trunk and limbs

    G. Other manifestations: arthralgia, thrombophlebitis, central nerve system (CNS) problems, erythema nodosum

III. Treatment

    No specific treatment available

Pemphigus Vulgaris

  I. Etiology

    Unknown

 II. Signs and symptoms

    A. It occurs during middle age or beyond.

    B. This systemic skin disease may be confined to the mouth for months before it appears elsewhere.

    C. Systemic symptoms of malaise, loss of appetite, and weight loss are often present.

D. Oral manifestations consist of painful ulcerations of various sizes that have a ragged border and are covered by a white or blood-tinged exudate.

E. Lesions may extend onto the lip and be covered by crusts.

F. Most helpful test in differential diagnosis is biopsy of an intact fresh lesion.

III. Treatment and prognosis

   A. Systemic corticosteroids

   B. High mortality rate in untreated patients.

Stevens-Johnson Syndrome

Stevens-Johnson syndrome is a severe form of erythema multiforme with mucous membrane involvement (see Ch. 7).

Acute Necrotizing Ulcerative Gingivitis (Trenchmouth, Vincent's Infection)

I. Etiology

   A. A fusiform bacillus and a spirochete (*Borrelia vincentii*) are usually present in large numbers in a symbiotic relationship. Both of these organisms, however, are present in moderate concentrations in other oral cavity diseases.[7]

   B. Other factors include poor oral hygiene and a decreased resistance to infections.

II. Signs and symptoms

   A. Occurs most commonly in the age range 15 to 35 years

   B. Painful, hyperemic gingiva

   C. Sharply punched-out erosions of the interdental papillae. Papillae and gingiva bleed when touched and are covered by a gray, necrotic pseudomembrane.

   D. Often begins as an isolated focus of infection and rapidly spreads to involve the entire gingival margins.

   E. Fetid odor to breath

   F. Metallic taste

   G. Inability to eat because of pain and bleeding

   H. Headache, malaise, and low grade fever often

   I. Cervical adenopathy usually

III. Treatment

   A. Hydrogen peroxide mouthwash

   B. Systemic antibiotics: penicillin if not allergic

   C. Superficial débridement of the necrotic tissue improves oral hygiene.

  D. Recontouring of gingival papillae under the direction of a dentist may
     be necessary.

Erosive Lichen Planus

  I. Etiology
     Unknown
 II. Signs and symptoms
     A. Irregularly shaped erosions and ulcerations located on the buccal mu-
        cosa, lips, tongue, and palate
     B. Painful
     C. Often associated with nonpainful leukoplakia in a lacy pattern which
        is often seen on the border of the eroded areas
     D. Often associated with pruritic flat-tipped papules located on the flexor
        surfaces of the wrists and forearm, the inner aspects of the knees and
        thigh, and the sacrum
     E. Sometimes associated with diabetes mellitus
III. Diagnosis
     Biopsy of the lesion shows a characteristic histologic pattern.
 IV. Treatment and prognosis
     A. No specific treatment is very effective.
     B. Spontaneous regression may occur.
     C. Corticosteroid lozenges or systemic corticosteroids may be helpful in
        severe cases.
     D. Rare cases of malignant transformation have been reported.

Syphilis

  I. Etiology
     Treponema pallidum
 II. Primary stage
     A. Develops at site of inoculation approximately 3 weeks after contact
     B. The intraoral chancre covered by a gray membrane is an ulcerated,
        mildly painful lesion found most frequently on the lips, tongue, and
        tonsils.
     C. Darkfield examination is not helpful because *Treponema microdentium*
        is often present in the saliva of nonsyphilitic individuals.
     D. The chancre is highly infectious.
     E. Serology may not be positive at this early stage of disease.
III. Secondary stage
     A. Begins about 6 weeks after the primary eruption
     B. Diffuse skin eruptions

C. Oral lesions: multiple painless, grayish white plaques overlying an ulcerated surface and surrounded by erythema

D. Most often on tongue, gingiva, and buccal mucosa

E. Highly infectious

IV. Tertiary stage

    A. Occurs years after primary stage

    B. The gumma may occur in the oral cavity and most commonly involves the tongue and palate.

    C. The gumma is a firm nodular mass that may be mistaken for cancer.

    D. Atrophic or interstitial glossitis is another manifestation of tertiary syphilis.

V. Treatment

    Penicillin in varying doses and duration depending on stage of disease

Cancer

I. Etiology

    Alcohol and tobacco abuse are the major etiologic factors for oral cavity carcinoma.

II. Signs and symptoms

    A. Nonhealing painful erosions or ulcers appear.

    B. Common sites are the lateral portion of the tongue, floor of the mouth, and tonsils.

    C. Sore throat may be a symptom of cancer of the base of tongue (posterior one-third).

    D. Palpation is an important adjunct to inspection of the oral cavity. Base of tongue cancers may be most easily detected by palpation.

    E. Induration surrounding an ulcerated lesion is best detected by palpation.

    F. Leukoplakia (white plaque) may be a sign of cancer or may be caused by a completely benign condition.

    G. Metastasis to lymph nodes has occurred in 50% of cases by time of presentation.

III. Diagnosis

    A biopsy specimen of any suspicious oral cavity lesion is obtained.

IV. Treatment

    A. Depends on size and location of lesion

    B. Surgery, radiotherapy, or a combination of both modalities sometimes necessary

Nonulcerating Diseases

Candidiasis (Moniliasis, Thrush)

I. Etiology

    Infection is caused by *Candida albicans*, a yeast-like fungus.

II. Signs and symptoms

A. Occurs in young infants, in debilitated people, and after exposure to broad-spectrum antibiotics which destroy the normal organisms of the mouth and allow overgrowth of *Candida albicans*

B. White plaques on the buccal mucosa, palate, gingiva, and floor of the mouth

C. Occasionally involves the hypopharynx and esophagus and produces dysphagia

D. Stripping away the white plaque reveals a raw, bleeding surface.

III. Diagnosis

A. Plaque material can be examined microscopically in a potassium hydroxide preparation to show the typical hyphae with yeast buds.

B. Culture can also be performed.

IV. Treatment

A. Nystatin oral solution

B. Ketoconazole, an antifungal agent, may also be effective.

REFERENCES

1. Laskin DM: Etiology of the pain-dysfunction syndrome. JADA 79:147, 1969
2. Abrams RG, Josell SD: Common oral and dental emergencies and problems. Pediatr Clin North Am 29:681, 1982
3. Graykowski EA, Barile MF, Lee WB, Stanley HR: Recurrent aphthous stomatitis. JAMA 196:129, 1966
4. Graykowski EA, Kingman A: Double-blind trial of tetracycline in recurrent aphthous ulceration. J Oral Pathol 7:376, 1978
5. Von Vloten WA, Swart RNJ, Pot F: Topical acyclovir therapy in patients with recurrent orofacial herpes simplex infections. J Antimicrob Chemother 12:89, 1983
6. Straus SE, Seidlin M, Takiff H, et al: Oral acyclovir to suppress recurring herpes simplex virus infections in immunodeficient patients. Ann Intern Med 100:522, 1984
7. Shafer WG, Hine MK, Levy BM, Tomich CE: A Textbook of Oral Pathology. p. 778. WB Saunders, Philadelphia, 1983

Index ———————————————————————————————

Page numbers followed by f represent figures; those followed by t represent tables.

251